Live Out Loud

The Sisterhood *folios*:
LIVE OUT LOUD

© 2017 by CREATIVE PUBLISHING GROUP

Published by CREATIVE PUBLISHING GROUP

For any information regarding permission contact
info@creativepublishinggroup.com
www.creativepublishinggroup.com

ISBN 978-0-9958810-3-7

Printed in the United States of America
First publication, 2017.

Design: Amir Saarony

The Sisterhood *folios*

Live Out Loud

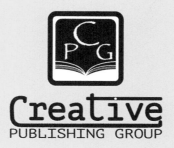

Creative
PUBLISHING GROUP

Acknowledgments

MICHELLE BIGGERS

I would like to acknowledge Dr. James and all the wonderful Specialists and nursing staff at the Hospital for Sick Children. I would also like to thank my son, Darrell Patrick Aidan Biggers, for saving my life and teaching me unconditional love.
Thank you and Blessings.

ADRIANE BREESE LLOYD

I would like to thank my husband Rene, who is my soulmate and has walked a very long journey with me. My daughters, Kiara and Olivia for loving me unconditionally. A very special thank you to Gyrga Andreev in Canberra, Australia, another Twinless Twin... who saved my life the first year. This story is dedicated to my beautiful twin sister Diana and all of the other Twinless Twins in this world.

LUCIA COLANGELO

To my sons, Jesse and Marco dreams may inspire me but You create my world.

SONIA COMMISSO

This book is dedicated to: My daughter Celia for giving me my rude "awakening" in my beautiful life! To my family and friends whose patience, kindness and love helped me through my journey. A special thank you to my mother who went to Portugal to pray to our Lady of Fatima for my daughter.

MARLA DAVID

I would like to thank all my friends and family who have supported me along my journey, in whatever capacity, whether you are aware of it or not. I would also like to thank Carol Starr Taylor for giving me the opportunity to have my voice heard - that I not die with anything left in me! I would also like to thank my birth mother for giving me life, and my parents for raising me with enough wisdom and wherewithal to be able to convey to others, the message I carry inside. Finally, I would like to thank the Sunshine.

LAUREN DICKSON

First of all, I would like to thank Carol Starr Taylor for this incredible opportunity! Writing has always been a passion of mine which I had been yearning to explore, and the idea of getting published and hopefully making a positive impact on the lives of the readers, is a feeling for which there are hardly words. It has been a struggle for me to look back on the heartache and pain of my past, and with her guidance I have strived to express my emotions and outlook. I would also like to thank my Mom. She has been through too many obstacles in her life, yet has remained a fighter and has always made her family her main priority. We may not always see eye to eye, but I don't know what I would do without her. Lastly, I would like to thank God. I don't always understand God's plan for my life, but I have learned to trust in him, and trust the timing of my life. It has been by God's grace that I am the fierce warrior that I am, and for that I will be forever grateful.

JENNIFER FEBEL

I want to say thank you to my husband and best friend, Brian, for supporting me on my journey and for always believing in me. And thank you to my clients – though you come to me for healing it is I who am truly healed for having walked your Journey with you.

ANDREA JUDIT
I would like to thank my parents for their ongoing loving support and putting up with me for 10 months while I was homeless, depressed and beside myself. Greatest thanks to my unbelievably supportive children Nicole and David and their spouses, who were there for me in the hardest times. I would also like to thank The Sisterhood *folios* and Carol Starr Taylor for this wonderful project she and her team have put together.

SAMANTHA KING
For Jeremy, Penny and Max. You guys inspire me, drive me crazy and hold me up each and every day. I couldn't do any of it without each little something that only each of you can bring to my day. For my closest fempreneurs. You are some of the strongest women I know. Your guidance, mentorship and unconditional support have brought me to tears on more than one occasion. You're some of the most giving and inspiring women I know, and I do what I do knowing that women like you are there to help me as we take the conversation to the next level. I am so lucky to know each and every one of you. You know who you are.

NATASHA KOSS
I would like to thank my husband, mother, father, sister and those who believe in me and my ability to write with freedom and raw emotion. Most of all I thank my daughter who teaches me everyday what it means to be alive and living.

GWENDA LAMBERT
Much love and gratitude to those who listened: Karen, Deb, Tracey, Carol, Geri, 240 Crew (Tony, Enzo, Mireille, Sally, Sarah and Fil) and my healing team: Leslie and Liz at Yoga Grove, Janet, Victoria, Marija, Miyako and Maureen.

MICHELLE MAIN

Thank you to my beautiful son Carson for choosing me to be your mom. You are such a blessing. You are the light of my life and I love you Always and Forever with all my heart. To my husband who loved me even when I didn't deserve it and put up with me for 28 years. I will always love you. To my mom for showing me what a strong woman is and for being by my side always. You were the first person I ever wrote I love you Always and Forever. To my dad, thank you for being the first man in my life. My protector. My Angel. I miss you and love you Always and Forever.

CLAUDINE PEREIRA

I would like to thank my advisory board who gave their stamp of approval on this chapter. The Pink Bench crew I couldn't do this without you!

PETRA REISS WILSON

I would like to thank all who have helped in my life journey especially my husband Bradley who has given me unconditional love and support and my father and mother who gave me a strong personality. Love to all.

SARAH SHAKESPEARE

I would like to thank my parents Trescott and Christine Powell for helping me see that anything was possible in life. Their love of life was inspirational and I continue to live my life with the tools that they instilled in me as a child. Till we meet again xo.

CAROL STARR TAYLOR

I dedicate this book to my Matriarch, the Angels from which I came from. You taught me unconditional love, strength and courage. To my Great Grandmother Rachel, Grandmothers Anne (Sarah) and Esther and to my Mother Doreen. To the

Wonderful Sister Authors in this book that took a chance, stepped out of their comfort zone and dug deep to inspire. To Heidi Allen, who graced our book with the foreword. To the Sisterhood all over the world that continue to inspire and are inspired through your voice being heard. Finally, to my 3 Children, who are my why and legacy. I am proud of each and every one of you.

AMY STOCKWELL
To my children who gave me a reason and stopped me from running from myself! To Carrol Campbell for all the mentoring and learning, and to my Mom for all the wise quotes I keep in my thoughts at all times.

TERESA URSINI
Thank you Robert for all your unconditional love, respect, strength and inspiration. My Parents for their unconditional love, wisdom and family values. To Alan Frew thank you for the lyrics/music and inspiration. Thank you to special family & friends too many to mention. To Carol Starr Taylor, thank you for the opportunity to be part of the Sisterhood *folios*.

GILLIAN JOY WHYATT
I would like Thank my mom and dad for giving me life and for my Dad who was and will always be my hero! To my beautiful daughters who are growing into young women who are on their own journeys and writing their own stories. Also I want to thank those who are not mentioned but you know who you are who played a part in this Journey of mine! Thank you, I love you!

TABLE OF CONTENTS

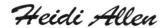

Foreword

When I was asked to write the foreword for The Sisterhood *f*olios: Live Out Loud, I felt honored. It immediately made me think about what it means to be a part of a group; an alliance; a community. For me I've always had a large circle of friends. Young companions and older friends; some are really successful while others are starving artists. And of course, I've got a few lost souls in my group as well.

These connections are supportive, caring and passionate, and filled with love. When I think about it, my beautiful friendships are my most cherished collections. It is within these relationships that we are able to flourish and lead a positive life.

I feel it comes from my belief that everyone comes into our life for a reason, a season, or a lifetime. Each and every soul union is needed and embraced.

When a 'Reason Friend' walks into your life, these bonds become incredibly important. They are the allies granted to us to guide and teach the lessons we need to learn. These teachings can sometimes be hard and emotionally painful, but they make us very aware of how we need to change, grow and succeed. Embrace these magnificent friendships and learn to let go when you have absorbed what you need. A new experience will be right around the corner.

The next incredible connection is the 'Season Friend'. I always love these friends because we unconsciously call them into our life. These amazing folks appear when we crave a particular personality or experience. They are the unexpected whirlwind relationship that reminds us who we are or who we want to be. The meetings are short-term and exhilarating when they happen. They spark something within and become great reminders in life when we need it.

A 'Lifetime Friend' is a glorious gift we are bequeathed. Their unconditional love and support helps build the foundation of our lives. They are responsible for the lifelong lessons we are to learn and accept. These will always be the dearest people in our lives that make everything worthwhile. Cherish and love these friendships and they will never let you down.

It is these positive unions that helped me found the Positive People Army; a movement of like-minded people who want to share their stories, support each other and spread positive energy. It is a community focused on inspiring and motivating each other to become better versions of themselves. The army's only goal is to remind each and every one of us that there is good in every situation, and possibility in every person.

Skimming the pages of The Sisterhood ƒolios: Live Out Loud, I found some of the narratives describing heartwarming relationships, heartache, and journeys of self-discovery created by interactions with people brought into our lives; something very similar to the Army's mission.

Living out loud can mean something to one person and create a completely different scenario to someone else. Yet, no matter what the circumstance, as long as we embrace true authenticity and the people that make our lives possible we will always succeed!

Thank you Carol for bringing together the incredible women in this book. Their stories teach us all that a sisterhood is necessary and truly powerful.

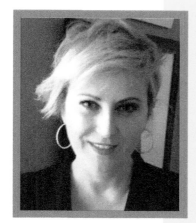

Heidi Allen began her journey as a successful wedding photographer but knew she was supposed to be doing something bigger. Determined to make her mark and make a difference, her next careers: wedding gown store owner, lifestyle editor for a popular wedding magazine, co-host for a morning drive radio show—were the same. After working as a TV host, she settled on the Marilyn Denis Show as a makeover producer helping women transform their lives.
All of a sudden something changed within her. She realized she was meant to motivate and inspire people on a larger level. The Positive People Army movement began. Heidi Allen is also a regular contributor to The Huffington Post.

Carol Starr Taylor

Mamma Mia

Mommy, Mom, Ma, Mum, Mamma, Mamman, Madre, Mami, Ema, Mother, Ahm, Mae, Mor, Mama, Mana, whatever you call yours, we have all had one—whether you knew her or not. The word itself cannot be uttered without some emotion attached to it. The term, "mother" is loaded with thoughts, feelings, and emotions. At least it is for me.

One thing I can ascertain is that most of us are never indifferent about our mothers. Love them or hate them, there really isn't anything in between. What was your experience with your mother? What IS a mother exactly? Is she the one who gave birth to you or the one that raised you? Is she both? How do you truly feel about your mother?

As a society, we are conditioned that all mothers should be these nurturing, loving, gentle, caring, women. We are force-fed this ideology through social media, Hallmark holidays, television sitcoms, and movies. We have a utopian view of how amazing our mothers are and how our relationships should be with them. Anything else falling short of this is an anomaly, total and utter dysfunction. However, in reality it can be, and in many cases is, less than exemplary to say the least. Dysfunctional relationships with our mothers

14

tend to be more common than we are led to believe. Many of us are afraid to admit that, at least publicly. It somehow makes us a "bad person" that we do not like, love, or do not have a relationship with our mothers. Please do not confuse loyalty and obligation with love. It is not the same thing. It isn't easy to come to terms with such a convoluted relationship and realize that there possibly was, or is, no love there.

> "Probably there is nothing in human nature more resonant with charges than the flow of energy between two biologically alike bodies, one of which has lain in amniotic bliss inside the other, one of which has labored to give birth to the other. The materials are here for the deepest mutuality and the most painful estrangement."
> ~ Adrienne Rich of Woman Born: Motherhood
>   as Experience and Institution

A plethora of books, articles, paintings, poems, movies, songs, and jokes have been about mothers and motherhood. Mothers are fixtures in our society and so prevalent. Under relationship status with our mothers it should read "it's complicated." For those of you that have a great relationship with your mother, was it always so? Men, do you dote on or have a devoted mother or have you been at odds?

Many of us have seen our mothers struggle in some way or another—emotionally, physically, financially, or all of the above. We have seen her strength, yet many of us use HER life experiences as a benchmark for our own of what we do NOT want to do, say or live. How many of you are horrified when you catch yourself saying something your mother would have said? I certainly have. As soon as I utter it, I'm dismayed and sometimes laugh that I just said that. From birth to death, the constant flow of energy that we spend thinking about our mothers is monumental. All the drama, arguments, celebrations, love, interactions, because of, and with our mothers seem to have a colossal impact in shaping our own personal world and who we have become.

So why am I bringing up mothers? Well, I know for sure that I can't write about my life without writing something about my mother. Also, from the chaotic relationship I have had with my mother throughout my childhood all the way to adulthood, there has been clarity and valuable life lessons I would like to bestow upon you in this chapter.

I can say that for the first 49 years of my life, it was like we were in the Tower of Babel, the story in the Old Testament. We spoke completely different life languages and neither one of us understood the other.

We just didn't "get one another."

Indifference is definitely not what I experienced with my mother. Mothers and daughters have a totally different dynamic than mothers and sons.

> "It is one of the oldest mothering cliches in the book. But the idea of mothers favoring their sons over their daughters could be much more than just a stereotype, a poll suggests. And though they may be loath to admit it, mothers really do have favorites, it found. They are more likely to describe their sons as 'funny', 'cheeky', 'playful' and 'loving'.
>
> But when it comes to their daughters they are far more critical – believing them to be more 'stroppy',

'argumentative' and 'serious', according to the study
by parenting website Netmums.

The survey... found that mothers were twice as likely to
be critical of their daughters than sons – 21 per cent
compared to 11.5 per cent... Women in particular seem
to carry the feelings of parental disapproval and negative
typing into their adulthood...Mothers were more likely to
attribute positive personality traits to their sons than
their daughters"
~Laura Clark, Daily Mail (UK) October 5 and 6, 2010

I ached for her to love me. She just couldn't. I longed for her acceptance all through my childhood and it never came. Cold, shrill, no hugs, no affection of any kind. Constant criticism. I was starved. Starved from a mother's love actually sounds absurd, considering the circumstances of a planned pregnancy and birth.

Malnourished is how I can describe the relationship between my mother and me. No mother would ever admit publicly she hates her child, especially in a closed knit cultural demographic—it is unfathomable. But, you just know it. You sense it. I felt it each and every day of my life.

I knew what I was missing, because my grandmother loved me unconditionally. I would often question to myself, why my mother can't be like her mother and show me love. A grand-mother's love is amazing and I was so blessed that I had had that, but it is not the same as the love from your own mother. I wanted my mother to think I was the best, her first born. To think I was talented. To acknowledge I was beautiful. No. None of this came. No matter what I did to try and please her. I never measured up. I was too fat, too skinny at times, looked like my dad, not too smart, a failure and not pretty. To HER. I clearly wasn't her favorite. Her views about me shaped me into the woman I was to become. It took years, with much introspection, work, knowledge, poor choices, and learning experiences to undo the damage that was created. I felt inconsequential.

I totally gave up. I stopped trying to seek her approval that I knew would never come. I felt that I was unlovable and rejected by my own mother. What does that do to a person? Anger and rage instead of love filled my heart. Hate and I mean an outright loathing for her very existence filled my body and soul for her, starting in my early teenage years. That disdain engulfed me until I was 49. A real vicious cycle, I HATED MYSELF FOR HATING HER. She didn't understand me, but I did understand her. However, my empathy towards her was clouded by disappointment and hatred. Never indifference. I really couldn't comprehend a woman who was so kind, sweet, and loved by all who met her and knew her; how could she be like this to me? What did I do to deserve this? I wasn't asked to be born. By no fault of my own, I was born. But by my own fault, I became a complete BITCH toward her. It was out of character for me with anyone else. I just couldn't help it, but I was always loyal to her. I guess it was a culmination of a lifetime of incidents that turned me to become that way with her. I had always felt guilty about that. I didn't like myself for behaving that way.

I always desired that amazing mother-daughter "thing" that others had or I perceived they had.

My parents finally divorced when my mother was 49, but not by her initiative. How many times in my childhood did I pray for that to happen? I was consumed with those thoughts as a child and plagued with the question in my mind: who would I choose to live with, Mr. Bad or Mrs. Worse? My position oscillated, depending on the day. Well, I didn't need to choose, because I was already grown up, 28, and married to, at that time, my second husband, the absolute love of my life.

I don't think it matters how old you are when your parents have that family meeting to let you know that they are splitting up. It shocks your very existence. As much as I wished it as a child, I hadn't really thought through what impact it would have on me. It pulled the rug out from under my feet. After 30 years of marriage, a couple of businesses together, three children, and at that time one grandchild from my sister, this was earth shattering news to say the least. They didn't get into details about what finally broke them, other than "too much has happened in 30 years." I didn't understand it then, but I did "get it" 20 years later in my own marriage.

Having said all of this, my observations of my mother certainly made an impact on me since my parents' separation and divorce. They were her actions that she made for her own life and weren't intended to be teachable moments for me. But, they were. What I found was, contrary to my own belief, that she was a remarkable woman. She had a silent roar. She was a fighter, being single after only knowing my father from age 18 to alone at age 49. Yes, he dumped her. After all those years, treating her as he did, he finally let her go.

Out into the world like a scared lion cub, she emerged as a lioness. She rebuilt her life, that she carved and created for herself that she eventually loved. Yes, life can start at 50.

Then life throws another curve ball. My mother got sick. A long debilitating illness that she fought so hard, for seven years until I saw her take her last breath at the young age of 73.

Three years' prior, my mother and I made a magical break-through. She contracted pneumonia and was deathly ill at that time. The doctors in the hospital didn't think she was going to make it. Day and night I was at the hospital. Taking care of her, advocating for her. Out of loyalty, of course.

I don't know if it was because of me being the first born or my personality, but I was the one saddled with the responsibility to talk to her about her possible death. The tough discussion I had to have with her with regard to her unplanned funeral and her wishes. I saw her fight. I witnessed her resilience. Sitting at the edge of her hospital bed, we had THAT moment. The moment that I had spent my whole life pining for.

I sat at her hospital bedside and held her hand. She held mine. I said softly but forthrightly, "Mom, do you not think it is interesting, that the kid you've hated your whole life, is the one taking care of you, now?"

I wasn't angry. I was deeply sad. I said it quite matter of fact-like. She gripped my hand firmly and softly answered, "I know." She continued, "I never meant to be like that to you. It came out all the time because I was angry. I was under your father's thumb. I felt trapped. You didn't make it easy for us, either. You really are a good daughter. A good person. Carol, I want you to know that you are beautiful." And for the first time, in, I can't ever remember, she told me she loved me. We both had tears in our eyes. Finally, we spoke the same language! At that very moment, time stood still. It was a new age. A new beginning for us. All of the past resentments and anger vanished, replaced with mutual respect and, yes, love.

> "I do not think there's anything more important than making peace before it is too late. And it almost always falls to the child to try to move toward the parent."
> ~ Jane Fonda

I do not think that if I hadn't been so candid that day, that moment, that the relationship wouldn't have flourished as it did. Sometimes you need to address things head on; it may not be pleasant but better to discuss than keep silent. I hadn't planned to express myself, it just came out in the moment.

All those lost years, living in absolute misery. It is a tragedy that it takes being so close to death to finally have an epiphany. All those missed opportunities, to say the things that should have been said long ago. This demonstrates how communication of less than five minutes could have indeed changed both of our lives. The lesson, of course, is to not live with regret and never leave this life with things left unsaid.

My mother and I had three years of closeness. For that I am forever grateful. We talked about everything. I was a confidant for the secrets of her marriage to my father, and the lies that had to be told in order to stay married.

I witnessed her rapid decline. Her fight. Her strength. Her struggle. I was faced with probably the most difficult things I have ever had to endure. My mother's condition was rapidly becoming unstable. I was alone in the room with her until the

ICU team joined us. They presented the choices to me for the next plan of action. I quickly called my sister on the phone, who was delayed in her arrival. I then had to have the agonizing undertaking to question my mother, slowly, one last time.

"Mom, they can take you up to ICU now and intubate you again, but they are not sure if this will help, or, they can make you comfortable and you will pass away." I felt like I was choking. I was softly crying, of course, as to make sure I received a response from her.

As this was all unfolding, I am screaming to myself inside. I was silently freaking out. Saying to myself... Carol don't lose it. Keep it together. Be strong. You need to be there for Mom. Stop crying. STOP Crying. This is her honor, to live with dignity and to die with dignity. YOU owe her that.

I waited silently. She then responded with "yes" to both.

I was holding back the tears as much as I could. An unknown surge of strength engulfed me. I said, "Mom, PLEASE, (I urged), you need to be clear, you can ONLY choose one, and I can't and won't make the decision for you. You need to choose. You are in charge. Do you want to go to ICU or the hospital will make you comfortable? You WILL pass away."

She uttered with her labored breathing, "I can't live like this anymore."

It was her choice to be had and hers alone.

My mother demonstrated her ultimate strength and determination as she waited 14 hours until all three of her children were at her bedside. Her last breath. The gut wrenching agony I felt as she lay in her hospital bed in silence, in her final peace. The wound of the invisible umbilical that was ripped from my very soul will never fully close. I was now part of the "I Lost My Mother Too" club.

I had thought that my father's death was utterly devastating. Shocking most certainly. Horrendous absolutely. That loss indescribable. A different sense of emptiness consumes me, as I feel the loss of my mother. Not the same. Far worse than can be fathomed. To lose a mother, the woman who carried me, hated me, and then loved me.

As life has gone on, and I experienced joys and sorrow, there has been and will always be a deafening silence. No one to call. No one who understands me and accepts me unconditionally. The sudden realization that I was part of the worst club of them all. THE ORPHAN CLUB.

BOOM! IT HIT ME! The moment I realized when I finally became an adult. To live a life with no parental guidance. Even when you do not ask them for advice, you know they are there, waiting in the wings, to pick you up when you are down. Not anymore. No unconditional love from the ones that knew you from the very beginning of time. Going it all alone, and somehow standing strong.

What have I learned from all of this? A few inspirations that I would like to share with you:

1) Your parents did the best they could. Now as an adult, I realize they never told me how many nights they cried. How many days they suffered in silence with smiles on their faces as we do every day. How they faced challenges and demons within themselves and overcame the struggles that faced them in their daily lives. What their marriage really looked

like behind closed doors and what secrets they kept to their graves. What it was like to each be single and find other partners, as so many of us do each and every day. We never looked at them as people, as a man and a woman; they were just our parents.

2) Relationships can mend and we can live with no regrets.

3) It is never too late for anything.

Things my mother taught me that I wish she hadn't:

To take abuse
To be dependent
To worry
To live being frightened
To stay silent
To settle for less than deserved
To morph your life to your partner's life
To give up all your hopes and dreams
To keep secrets and tell lies to cover up
To stay in an unhappy relationship
To have no self-love
To have no self-esteem
To have no self-worth

Things my mother thought me that I'm glad she did:

To be a fighter
It is never too late to start your life over
It is never too late to rebuild relationships
Charity
To be humble
Education is important

Loyalty
Honesty
Hard Work
Cultivate your own friends (she did this later in life)
Be resilient
Forgiveness
Kindness
Strength

And finally, I think the most poignant lesson is that, there comes a time in our lives where we need to take responsibility for our own actions and stop blaming our parents. To stop being bitter over decisions that they made, which affected our lives that we aren't happy about. To understand that we can change our path. That we are the architects of our own lives. It is not your parents' fault things aren't going your way. It is also not your parents that accomplished all the amazing things you have achieved. Know that we have the ability to overcome the chaos of our pasts and pave the way for our glorious future with clarity.

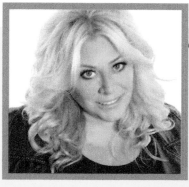

Carol Starr Taylor is the Founder of Creative Publishing Group, Writing Coach, Certified Life Coach, NLP Practitioner, International Bestselling Author of the book Life In Pieces – From Chaos to Clarity, Inspirational Speaker, Soulprenuer, and the Founder of The Travelling Sisterhood. She has appeared on TV, Radio, Podcasts, and has been featured in numerous articles. Her passion is to inspire and help facilitate the personal growth of others within themselves and with each other.

Michelle Biggers

The Miracle of Love

He was sitting outside the back door on the stoop, with his little hands set gently on his knees... in a lotus position, with sticks of gathered wood laying at his delicate five-year-old feet.

I could not believe what I was seeing as a warm rush of love and gratitude enveloped me.

I ran to get my phone to take a picture of this incredible sight! At five years of age, this gift of a child, has more connection and communication with God, our Creator and universe, than I could ever hope to have.

While living in a hell of depression and anxiety, God had decided to give me one last lifeline. I didn't know it at the time, but this event would alter the course of my life, the way I thought, and how I perceived myself, and others around me. Ten years ago, I was blessed with a miracle that saved me from an existence of hopelessness and constant suffering. No one else could do this for me. I was called upon to stand on my own and become responsible, finally, for who I was.

I felt like the earth had opened up and swallowed me whole. I lay in bed for days at a time; it was painful just to get up to go and relieve myself. My thoughts were dark and racing as I isolated from my children, Pete, my estranged husband, and anyone else that tried to be a part of my world.

I had lost weight and was only 98 pounds. I tried to eat but as soon as the food hit my mouth, I started to gag. I did not want to live, but was too afraid to die.

Depression is a hell that no one can understand, unless you have experienced it yourself. Well-meaning family members and friends would try to empathize, but words fell onto deaf ears, as though they had not been spoken at all. At times I had been hospitalized. It could be that I never got over the death of my daughter, Genevieve, at her birth, or that I was a failure at my third marriage, that I never felt I belonged, or that I was good enough. The doctors said Genevieve's death was unexplainable. They also told me never to get pregnant again because I would die, the baby would die - or both.

Depression was my friend on and off for years. This was all I knew. I buried myself into an abyss of hopelessness and despair for months at a time. I went unmedicated, even unaware of the suffering I was inflicting on my family, and most of all, myself.

I had recently moved back from out of province, leaving behind a destructive marriage in a twenty-year relationship with a man I desperately loved. It hurt that this love was not reciprocated the way I needed it to be. I was self-medicating to stuff down the pain as we tried to co-parent, renting our separate units in a duplex. It was not working well.

I forced myself to accept an offer from a friend, for a sales and marketing position. I met Krissy at the office and we quickly became friends. I started to see an older gentleman that would take me out once a month. I felt at least someone was noticing me in a good way. Work was hard, but kept me from rotting away in my bed, and I seemed to become one of the best on the team. I felt this was because I could lose myself in a different world, I could be someone else... someone that had a different name, and was happy and successful. This worked while I was in the office, but the moment I left for home, the real me resurfaced with a rage, with all the dark horrors, never relenting, ceaseless, shrieking cries; my other reality.

Still self-medicating, with my new gentleman friend I found out I was pregnant. I was shocked and knew that I needed to start caring for myself if I was going to get through this pregnancy alive, or had any chance of carrying the baby.

The gentleman disappeared when I shared the news. I was again rejected and not good enough. Why was it, other women could maintain a marriage, have happy relationships, be financially stable, but every time I attempted to get my life together, it would fall apart? What was their secret? The journey over the next year would finally teach me what that secret was. As I sat with legs up at my office desk, chatting with my co-workers, I felt a gush of liquid... uh oh, I can't do this now! I'm way too early to give birth today! I wheeled myself into the bathroom to confirm that I was bleeding. My first reaction was panic, then calm, as I realized that this was going to happen, regardless of whether or not I wanted it to, or if I was ready for it. At this moment, all I thought of was not losing another child. I could not deal with another death.

Krissy calmed me as I called Pete to take me to the hospital. The office was excited, but very careful with me as two office chairs were wheeled to the door - me sitting on one and my feet up on the other. I did not want to have this baby on the floor, as I had miscarried this way at home one other time.

Pete arrived, shaken, but fully prepared for the familiar hospital run. He slowly wheeled me out and lifted me into the car, ensuring I was in the back seat with my legs elevated. I could not hold back the tears as I knew both myself and my baby were in danger.

We arrived at the closest hospital and were immediately rushed into the delivery room. Everything happened so quickly. I was over 8 weeks early and had been as sick-as-a-dog, vomiting, throughout the whole pregnancy.

I was told they needed to do an emergency C-section. All of my other children, accept the first, were delivered naturally and without pain medication, so I was beside myself, upset and confused with the emergency C-section. I tried to be brave, understanding they needed to get the baby out immediately.

The doctors scrubbed up and within minutes I was frozen and cut open. Out came the tiniest, most frail looking baby; I waited for him to cry, but didn't hear a sound. Was he alive? Why couldn't I hold him? Where were they taking him? I tried to get answers but they were too busy stitching me up and taking care of the baby to answer me. Maybe they didn't know if he would live? I was in anguish, not knowing what was happening to him.

They quickly took him and placed him into an incubator. The doctors said that he needed to be sent to a Level-3 care facility. He was extremely jaundiced, had a small head, and only weighed two pounds. I was shaken and confused.

Arrangements were being made to take him to another hospital. It felt as though time stopped. I was not able to see him or hold him. I was put to rest in another room and waited, frightened and anxious to know if he was going to make it. "Dear God, please let my baby be okay."

The doctor came into the room and informed me that the baby was now in transit. "I have to follow him," I declared. The nurse implored that I stay and rest as I was not well. I didn't care. All I could think of was my little one. I had to be with him, he needed me! Pete wheeled me out, then carried me to the car and away we went for the hour-long journey to a hospital in another city. When we arrived my son was not there! I broke down, furious, more perplexed and desperate than before. Where was my child? Why was I not told? The nurse insisted that I needed medical attention and wanted to admit me for doctors' care. I could not. Why didn't they understand that I had to be with my baby? He had been moved again, this time to the Hospital for Sick Children (HSC).

Pete, again, carried me back to the car and traveled an hour to find my son at the HSC where we were told he had suffered from two seizures since birth, and had been admitted to Intensive care. I was angry! Why had they taken so long to get him here? Why did they not bring him here in the first place?

I was furious, scared, and processing emotions I didn't even know. I needed to blame someone for this incompetency! I was his mother and had every right to be with him, protect him, and know what was going on!

We finally got to see him. I had still not heard him cry. As I was wheeled into his room, there was a crowd of doctors and nurses around him, tending to his every need. I saw his frail, tiny, two-pound body, lying on his tummy, blind-folded, with tubes and wires coming from what seemed every part of his body. He was alive! We were told about the life-support systems he was attached to, but it went in one ear and out the other. I remember them saying there was a "pick-line" to his heart. He was completely helpless and I felt like it should have been me lying there instead of him. My innocent little baby, so alone and not able to feel the warmth of me, the scent of me. He needed his mother and I needed for him to know how much he was loved and wanted.

I started fervently praying for him. After the initial visit with the baby, the doctors asked us to please follow them into a separate room. I knew they were going to let us know what was wrong with him. The doctor started to list off a barrage of incomprehensible complications that he was suffering from. Sacral dimple, jaundice, and 12 other medical terms. The words that I dreaded came next. "He will never see, hear, walk, talk or speak. Prepare yourself to let him go."

Those words sunk into me with a thud, a black heaviness which defies description. I fought not to fall back into that black hellish hole where I would drown. I stayed focused on him and thought of nothing and no-one else, a complete place of unawareness and oblivion. Pete turned to me, then back to look at the doctors, then clearly stated, "It doesn't matter what is wrong with him. He will be like the rest of the other children. He will have brothers and sisters who love him. He will be a part of the family just the same." Now I remembered why I fell in love with this man.

This gave me a sense of comfort. Nonetheless, we were told he would not make it. I was numbed. I had no awareness of myself, what day it was, or even realized the state of my own medical risk.

I felt as though I was on the edge of a canyon; one slip and I would lose him. I was not willing to allow this little person to die or suffer. After some initial grieving, I could not discern whether to pray for God to let him die without pain, or to pray for him to fight for his life. I did not know how to pray, or what to pray for.

I wheeled myself back into his room, just asking God to do His will and to give me the strength to accept what His will was. I got closer to his incubator, where he was lying face down, completely unaware of his surroundings or even of his life... unable to see me or hear me. I pushed as close to him as I could get and raised my baby finger up to the bubble and into his incubator. His tiny, feeble hand lifted up from his body and grabbed onto my finger and held it with all his feeble strength and might. I completely broke. I sobbed with tears of joy. This tiny little soul had felt my presence! He could not see me! He could not hear me! How did he know I was there for him? He did not let go and silently whispered to me, "My name is Darrell and I am here." I don't think I have ever felt joy like this in my life, neither before or since that moment.

God had shown me that there was hope!

During the days that followed I sat at his side, praying and singing, and believing he could hear me. I stared at his miniature fingers and toes, wanting to kiss and touch each one of them, but not being allowed to do so. How I longed for him to feel my touch.

Pete came to take me home briefly to change and get a break from sleeping in the hospital chair. Being all-consumed with hanging on to my baby and wanting him to be OK, it slowly occurred to me that I had other children to care for too. I was living in a fog, in a state of suspension, not being able to move forward, not being able to go back to change things, and somehow make this right.

After over-coming the 'self-talk' in my head, and knowing he would be watched, I went home to spend some time with them, all the while, anxious that I was away from my baby. I reassured the children that their little brother would get better and that I needed to continue to stay with him at the hospital. I comforted them saying I would be here as much as I could, and I would stay home that night.

I awoke the next morning screaming in pain from the razor-sharp feel of the sheets touching my skin. I could not move. The air hurt me, my clothes ravished me. I yelled for Pete; he lifted me with gentleness as I writhed in agony, and brought me to the nearest hospital. I was rushed into a room and put on an IV of two antibiotics and morphine. I was septic from infection, and next to death myself. After twelve hours of treatment I told the doctors I wanted to leave. I had to get to my baby.

The doctors said I must stay to continue treatment and monitoring. I said I was going to the HSC and would follow up with them there. I left against their recommendations. I never followed up. I lived, ate and breathed for Darrell.

I again sat by his side, talking to him, watching him breathe, watching his every wee movement in awe and anticipation. He still had not made any sound. I thought to myself that I would live here as long as it takes. Time seemed to stand still, I was living only in the moment, trying to let him know how much I loved him.

The daily rounds of the Doctors and the team were always one of the most important parts of the day. I would listen intently as they discussed Darrell's conditions and plan of treatment. I was thrilled when they said they were going to try to tube-feed him! I was asked to start pumping milk for him and to keep up a healthy supply, freezing what was not going to be used.

I lived between his bedside chair and the breast-pumping room for weeks. Every day, asking questions, speaking to the doctors, coming to know his nurses. I was saddened to see other precious little ones whose parents had never come in. I could not grasp how someone could have a child in NICU yet never be there by their side, never to even acknowledge the life they had created. That was heart-breaking.

After a month I was able to hold him!! I can remember as if it was yesterday! It was the brightest day since his birth! The only sounds he had made at this point were tiny little hiccups which I recorded on my phone.

I gently took him in my arms, careful not to disturb the wires andlines attached to his body and cried as I felt my baby in my arms. I held him close and kept him warm, putting him under my gown, beside my skin, so he could feel me, atune to my heartbeat, smell his mom, and begin to bond. I held him as long as they allowed, happy and content to have him close to my heart at last. I was even more joyful when his nurse said I could now change his diapers myself! Yayyyyy! I get to be a mom! There were further difficulties. Over the next three months, his weight would go up and then drop again. He had trouble with absorbing the breast milk at times. He went through thirteen blood transfusions and all the while, never seemed to complain; he was quietly fighting the best way he knew how.

On one of the rare occasions that I went home, I had an answer from God. I awoke at 3:00 a.m. and left the house to sit outside in contemplation. I needed for God to hear me. I yearned for some kind of indication that Darrell would make it home. It was gently sprinkling a warm, cleansing rain. Out of nowhere, all of a sudden, the skies opened up with a chorus of singing birds! It sounded like a song from heaven, with all different melodies, loudly singing, calling to me! I couldn't believe it! I had to phone my sister, two-thousand miles away, to ask her if this could really be happening. She laughed and gently, cautiously agreed, that this was a sign that God was taking care of Darrell. I knew deep in my heart that my baby was going to come home with me!

I held him daily, to my face, while I sang gently into his ear a lullaby that my grandfather used to sing to me, "tooruh lura lura... tooruh lura lie, toooruh lura lura, hush now, don't you cry." An old Irish lullaby. I would pray into his ears, knowing in my heart he would respond with hearing, never giving up hope.

Darrell was hypoglycemic, so every two hours the nurses pricked his miniature heel to check his blood sugar. They taught me how to do this while I was there. At times his blood sugar dropped dangerously low and we had to get breast milk into him immediately and it would rise again within minutes. It was touch-and-go for four months while we lived in NICU. After further testing, we were told he had Auditory Neuropathy – he could actually hear! Only at certain decibels, and with inconsistency, but he did have hearing! This was not the case when they first diagnosed him, but I knew better! Every day thereafter, my little boy fought and overcame the 14 complications of his birth. He opened his eyes and started to focus. He could see! He started to make sounds and eventually he cried! He could vocalize! One by one, Darrell came to rise above his challenges and come to life.

The doctor took me aside one day and said, "Your baby is saying to us, 'I'm not going anywhere, my name is Darrell and I will do things in my own time'!" This is how Darrell has lived his life. In his own time. I felt blessed when he told me the baby would not have pulled through without my love. You see, this is not a child that medically was meant to be. This precious child was a soul, a spirit born through Will. It is only through the will of God that he was able to fight for his life against all odds. It was only from LOVE that he was able to defy modern medicine's prognosis and live of his own will while doctors said he would not.

After three and a half months, I was able to take him for a real walk down the hall!! I was so happy! For the very first time, I could take him out of the NICU room and explore with him! It was the most wonderful time, as we walked up and down the hallway. His eyes slowly moved to take in the new surroundings. I loved the feeling of him in my arms, cuddling him and watching him take in a whole new world!

At times I thought he would never be able to leave this place, and would feel desperate when I had to leave him and come back over and over again. There were days when I was so sad and hurt because I missed my baby while traveling on the train, or when sleeping at home. I loved him so much and just wanted him to be with me, home, where I could smell him, nurse him, hold him and lovingly relish every moment with him. It is difficult to find words adequate enough to describe how it feels when you have to wait, day after day, week after week, month after month, to be able to go forward. Waiting for your child's life to be just OK.

When Darrell finally reached four pounds, they allowed me to bring him home! I was taught how to give him his injections which he needed every eight hours. I learned how to gently squeeze and pucker his meager thigh to find a place big enough to give him his lifesaving serum. The new challenge was just beginning and would continue for years ahead. Gratefully, humbly, finding joy in every task I needed to do to thank the Lord for this little life, I was living in gratitude.

Darrell walks, he talks, he sees perfectly, he runs, and has bionic hearing with the help of a Cochlear implant today. He has learned speech after eight years of AVT, Speech pathology, ASL, lip reading, visual aids, and Audiologists help. Physiotherapists and many other specialists have worked hard with us every day, month, week and year. We are hoping Darrell will be entering an English speaking school for the first time this fall! My gentleman friend has developed a close and caring relationship with his child and has changed his own life to become more grateful and aware, always there for Darrell.

One Christmas Eve, he drew pictures of all the family that would be arriving the next day for dinner. Every family member was a heart, drawn within a body. The heart was the person, not the body around it. When he showed me his picture of myself, it was incredible! He had used yellow and purple crayons; my body was purple, while I had yellow light streaming from my head, heart and hands into the rest of the page and upward to the sky. I almost dropped to my knees.

This child could see and had vision clearer and more complex than most humans ever reach. He saw people's auras and souls. My son, later that same evening, was found sitting outside in a lotus position, hands on his knees, eyes closed, in a deep state of meditation. I had never meditated in this position, always starting my morning ritual of silence and surrender while he was still sleeping, before all the children awoke. Where did he learn how to do this? How did my five-year-old know, and where was his mind traveling to while he was in this trance?

When Darrell was three, we visited a new Pediatrician once for a check-up. As we entered the room, the doctor was sitting, weary-looking, with her hands open facing upward on her lap. Darrell promptly toddled up to her and placed his hands upon hers. At once, she said, "He is a healer; he is gifted." This was unsolicited and an amazing thing to hear from an MD. This statement was confirmed as friends from within the community would visit and the ones that were unwell, remarked how Darrell would sit close beside them, holding onto them, and their pain would be taken away. Friends experiencing emotional challenges, or suffering from mental ailments, would also visit often as Darrell's loving, gentle touch would absorb their hurt or fears.

I now know that Darrell is gifted and in transcendence with the Creator. Darrell is a greater "seer" than me. This soul inside a tiny human has been born with purpose and great intent. This child is a profound healer and angel. He is total love. Every morning he awakens with the greatest of joy, just to be.

I live each day in grace, humility, and wonder at how I have come to be so blessed as to have the greatest opportunity and responsibility, to guide and nurture this divine spiritual person. I am in awe of God's miracle, and am one of the most grateful women on the earth for such an incredible, inexplicable gift to have been bestowed upon me, and the rest of the world.

This child saved me from the very death of my own soul, after years of depression and self-medicating. Never give up. Miracles do happen. I have learned from his precious, vibrant soul, what the secret is. The secret that all those 'other' happy people have found. The secret is unconditional love; to live each day in the moment, with deep gratitude, joy and faith, for that is all there is.

I know Darrell will be with me all my life, loving, teaching, and guiding me as a spiritual mentor, as much as I do him, as his mother. I know that miracles are real. His life is a miracle, as is mine. Every morning and night, I open and close my eyes, and surrender to life, as I have been shown what it truly means - to just love.

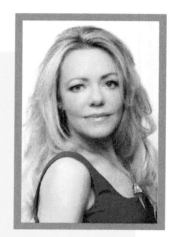

From a young age, **Michelle Biggers** has been blessed with the gifts of vision and healing. Michelle started teaching at the age of seventeen and opened a private school of the arts at age twenty-one. Throughout her journey of giving birth to seven children, and overcoming great challenges, she left the corporate world to open Whole Fitness Canada, for body, mind and soul. Michelle is a Certified Minister and Fitness Award winner, author, speaker and visionary.

Lucia Colangelo

My Vintage Collection

It had always been her gift to pair wines with her friends. From the time she was in her twenties and had discovered that not all wine was the strong, dark and heady homemade vino her Nonno (Grandfather) fermented in his garage in the fall, she had been intrigued with the wines of the world. Stored on homemade shelves in the cantina, the oak barrels filled with the potent vino that kept the family meals lively. Wine was the vitality that flowed through the roots of her family tree, each generation bringing its own distinction. But the origin, the beginning, the seed, was the same, the simple grape. The fruit that grew in clusters, bunched together, creating their own habitat, yet all linked together by the same vines and leaves, like families in her tree. Each ancestor creating its own bunch, yet their blood, their source of life, their connection was all bound together in a crazy, beautiful tangle of love, hate, betrayal, failure, success. Life.

The click of the antique lamp broke the silence. Its warm light casting a welcoming glow on the table set for five. It was a casual night, one to celebrate friendship; it had been a while since they were together. She had ordered the authentic, oven baked pizza from her favorite local Italian trattoria. Margherita:

the most simple, yet all agreed, the most delicious pizza, sweet ripe tomatoes, mozzarella fior di latte, fresh basil, salt, and olive oil. Giovanni would be delivering it at 9:00. That would give them enough time to enjoy one other, and the delicious salad she had prepared, bursting with different flavors, blended together in the colorful clay bowl that had been her Nonna's (Grandmother's). The sweet, juicy watermelon together with the ruby ripe tomatoes softened the spiciness of the arugula, the salty Mediterranean feta adding zing, a touch of olive oil, and tangy balsamic vinegar creating a euphoric taste. She turned to her wine cabinet, reminded of the quaint little shop in Venice. Crowded with second hand antiques, the beautiful workmanship of this one piece caught her eye, and she knew she had to bring it home. Now as she touched the warm wood she thought she could smell Venice and her mind got hazy with memories of the city that was home in her heart.

The first bottle was waiting to be placed on the table. She had opened it earlier, giving it a chance to release its unique aroma of vanilla, wood, spiciness, the color beautiful dark ruby, and its complexity showed its nature; big, bold, colorful, strong. Maleatis 2009 (Red) Greece. The wine she had chosen for Her. She closed her eyes and inhaled the earthy scent. Her mind went back years to grade nine, first day, first class, homeroom. Her eyes were immediately drawn to the pretty blonde girl sitting at the back of the room. Nervously she walked towards the empty desk behind the girl. She didn't realize until years later that it had been the stranger's aura that had drawn her. All she knew was that she must be a cool girl, already defying the rules by applying makeup at her desk. The wine filled her memories and she pictured her clearly in her mind. Sophia.

Sophia's Colors

The Angel sat fierce and powerful before her, his eyes like fire burning through to her soul. The horse he rode majestic, wild, his mane blowing like the flames flashing from the rider's eyes. He reached down and with a touch she was seated next to him. When he wrapped his arms around her, she felt both heat and cold, an indistinguishable element. Sophia felt, not heard, the words he whispered, 'never fear for I will always be with you'. That was the day the dreams began. A loved one would appear; a vision while she slept. They would tell her goodbye, the time had come for them to leave. Sophia would wake up to the sounds of grieving and the news that her nighttime visitor had passed. She was four years old.

Sophia awakened from the trance, stretching like the felines she connected with. Her earliest memory always made her smile; it chose to come often, but never at her request, a reminder of her gift. She looked around the home in which she had loving showcased her personality, simple, yet spiritual objects she had collected on her travels to Greece, Turkey, Paris and Italy. Her beautifully intricate table filled with candles, flowers, incense, and Buddha. The walls filled with meaningful canvas paintings, words she lived by. Shelves filled with books, pictures of family positioned carelessly yet artfully between them. On the dresser, books by Frankl, Byrne, Dyer, Murphy, her mentors.

Sophia thought back to a time when she was an innocent child, the memories brought on by the visit from the Angel. It had been a childhood filled with illness, yet the force that was her soul guided her towards her longing to live a life with a spirit so free, so voracious that it was to be the foundation of her blossoming spirituality. Her identity had always been connected to her culture, the mythical and ancient teachings a part of her faith.

But illness and darkness has a way of dimming the light of even the most devout. Her gifts became obscured by the grief of betrayal and loss. The star of her first marriage had been her daughter, the miracle that kept her from tumbling too deeply into the blackness. With her second marriage she had felt the promise of hope; he was the great love of her life. But her illness overcame her once again, when inflicted with the pain of extramarital affairs, financial crisis and losses. With her health perilously declining, the doctors unable to help, she received her earliest memory one night with an awakened understanding that only she could help herself. Reaching out to Spirit, she had rediscovered her soul, her gifts, and her purpose.

Her trip to Greece soon after had been the start of her journey to recovery. Stepping off the plane to the wondrous view of mountains stirred such emotion that she wept tears as salty as the seas that calmed her meditations. When a concerned passenger asked her why she was crying, she turned with joy and whispered, "I'm home." Her ancestors had reached out to her and she had opened her heart to them.

She would forever be grateful for the gifts she had been blessed with. She knew her suffering had led her to her purpose; to help others find their path. She mastered hypnotherapy, Reiki and life coaching. Her practice was fulfilling and powerful. And so Sophia found her faith and love again.

Realizing the time, Sophia stretched and headed towards her bathroom. A night filled with lovely wine and food was always a delight, but the four friends she would be sharing them with made it so much more. The harmony of their colorful souls mesmerized her every time. The colors floating above them teasing and laughing where only visible to her eyes, but were felt by them all.

She placed Sophia's bottle in the center of the table.

Sighing, she reached for the next one, the one that had been the most difficult to choose. Domaine Gioulis 2015 Sofos (Greece), an overwrought, spicy wine with hints of cedar. It was better served aged. Unlike the uncertainty of life, which sometimes shocks us into realizing that we are not here forever, death is true and certain. We had both been in love with the same boy. It didn't matter that his grade eleven attitude would not let him look at a grade nine girl. We were rivals. Running to the smoking area at lunch to get a spot near where he hung out with his friends, we reached it breathless with hearts beating even faster at the sight of him. Two young girls blushing with love, we bonded in our misery. My dear friend Ella, a widow at an age where life was to have started giving back.

Ella's Rainbow

She was exhausted. Wonderfully exhilaratingly exhausted, it felt good to feel, even sore muscles. The bootcamp today had been a killer, but then the slaughter of 75 pounds of anguish would not be easy she smiled to herself. Her husband's death had filled her with emotions so heavy, she had been motionless beneath them. Gaining over 100 pounds in grief, the self-hate had followed. Ella turned off the steaming water and stepped on the scale. She looked with disbelief at the numbers, a couple more pounds down. The pride she felt was still unfamiliar, the long pain filled journey that left her a widow still intruding. Looking in the misty mirror she wiped it clean, seeing her reflection, and remembering all the times in the beginning she had watched it fog up again, her reflection fading, and been afraid that she too would disappear. Maybe she wanted to. The face that stared back at her confused her, the new contours promising familiarity. But it was her eyes that surprised her the most. They gazed at her, clear and focused. The red, swollen, angry eyes of past left behind. Ella had danced with death, not personally but in a way that had buried her spirit. Somehow, like the miracle of a rainbow after a storm, that spirit had caught a tiny flicker of life. Her heart recognizing its soul had beckoned it, intensifying the flame until she could no longer ignore it.

Ella had read that grief passed with time, but what if you were comfortable in the place that expected nothing from you? And so she fought to contain the flame. Then one day she accidentally connected to the look in her son's eyes, and there she saw a depth of sorrow that matched her own. He had lost her, too.

From that day on, she fed the fire in her soul by simply allowing herself to feel it. Every day she grew braver, stepping out of her misery slowly. And as she grew stronger she realized that it was okay to remember. Going to the places they loved together brought a sadness, but also a closeness to his memory. As Ella's memories became brighter so did the vision of her future. The day she realized that just because she was living her life, it didn't mean she was loving him less.

She brushed her hair, thinking how excited her friends would be to see her. Amazed at how in the short weeks since they had been together last she had continued to transform not only her appearance, but her life. She would show them her certificate.

She had worked hard, going to classes on the weekend and studying late into the night. She had passed with a 76 percent. The mark only a small indication of the confidence she had unveiled as her soul and her heart became united.

She placed the bottle on the table. Her attention now drawn to the pretty pastel label of the bright colored bottle. This one had been an easy choice. A whimsical wine bought just for fun, the name alone would provoke giggles from her friends, instant recognition. The woman attached to this bottle was everything the bubbly wine claimed to be: sparkly, flowery, fruity, slightly sweet, soft and luscious. Cupcake Moscato D'Asti. It was, in fact, the simple cupcake – chocolate, filled with fluffy white cream, like the center filling of her oldest friend's heart - that had brought the two of them together. She was the new kid in the class, grade four, when sweet Flora had offered her the cupcake. Their friendship had been iced with sweetness ever since. Flora, who was so kind-hearted that the negative souls were usually repelled, had succumbed to the greatest, the most dangerous emotion: love.

Flora's Flowers

Flora played with her paint-crusted hair and stared at the canvas. She had spent hours with a counselor in the beginning, training her mind not to judge herself, not to blame herself. She hadn't discovered her love of painting then, that slowly emerged as she came to realize that we only have control over how we respond to another's behavior, that we can't control their actions. As she started feeling better about her life, she joined her friend one night at a restaurant that was hosting a 'Paint Night'. When she picked up the brush for the first time and touched it to the canvas, filling the whiteness with color, something happened to her that she couldn't explain. She had found a way to communicate without words. No longer locked into the emotional chaos that had been her marriage, she had found her voice. Her paintings had started out for her as a way of expressing herself, to free her feelings from the restraints of addiction. And so began her journey, not only towards self-healing, but from the limitations that living with him had fixated in her mind.

As she painted and her talent emerged she started posting her artwork on social media. With every Like, comment of praise and support her confidence grew. She realized that she was worth more than the label she had been given by his dependence on substances. She had been the pawn that he used to mask his issues, his past, his weaknesses, to the world - and to himself. His drug of choice had really been self-destruction; the others were to lessen the pain of his struggles. Her mistake had been in believing in the two of them. Except for the birth of her daughters, her relationship with him had been filled with fear, self-doubt, embarrassment, and failure. When she got the courage to leave, her family and friends, by allowing her to grieve the loss of her marriage, and the man she had fallen in love with, had gifted her with the things she craved most: acceptance and respect. And then she didn't need to grieve anymore. She realized, that even though her paintings made others smile, what they were really saying was,' I am beautiful'. And that's all she really needed. The paintings were a reflection of her soul.

Then came the words, at first just simple descriptions of the paintings. Then about how she felt creating the work. What it meant to her, the feelings that were being created through colors. She started getting messages. The words made someone's day, gave them a little push towards a goal, made them smile. Flora sipped on the sugarless green tea she drank when working, thinking about how simple her blog had come about. And like the flowers in her paintings she grew with the warmth of love. Flora's blog was created as a way to merge her paintings, her words, and her new healthy style of living all in one. The pleasure that others got from reading it was like the icing on, well, a cupcake!

Away from the influence of negativity, she had found herself realizing that one of the hardest paths you will travel is the one that will benefit you the most. Trying to stay away from toxic people in your life that take the most from your heart, and being strong enough to say, 'I deserve more', not only to them but to yourself. She understood now that they not only want you to believe you're worthless, they believe that about themselves. If you really were worthless, you would be on the floor already, and they wouldn't like that, because that's where they want to drag you. So she had walked away from 'worthlessness', surrounded herself with 'worthiness', and redefined herself into 'worth more'.

She turned away from the canvas, sighing deeply, torn between wanting to finish the painting and get ready to meet her girlfriends for dinner. She would get ready, of course. They had been by her side throughout it all, throughout her marriage, where innocence was still the main character, and now in the current chapter of her journey. She had much to tell them. Last month she had gone to Paris on her own. It had been scary, exhilarating and liberating! She had felt beautiful and desired, sitting at cafes outside in the sunshine.

The pretty dresses she had bought for the trip perfect in their simplicity and sexiness. Men glanced with eyes filled with appreciation. She smiled back at them. And she smiled now.

She set Flora's wine next to the others. Her mind slowly emerging from the thoughts of Flora's amazing transformation, she turned next to the bottle commanding attention. Caviccioli, Lambrusco di Sorbara, Vigna del Cristo, Italy, 2014, this wine structured, vibrant, incredible texture, remarkable richness, with a luscious finish, zesty, and not too sweet. My dear friend Lilly, the only one of us still married. She had been in the same grade-four class with Flora and me. The tomboy with dark, wild, crazy curls that sizzled with the energy she powered even then. Her runway to success as business partner to her husband had been hard, but one she had catwalked her way through with eyes shut and hips swaying. She had pushed herself, but always found the top unreachable. Until she realized that the top was a place that we each created in our minds.

Lilly's Shiny Red Soles

Show a woman a Louboutin and her eyes will glaze over, her breathing will deepen. Are they really that beautiful? Or is it that they symbolize what we all desire; be successful, desirable, untamable, seductive, wealthy, and mysterious? A flip flop is more comfortable, it doesn't pinch, or strain, but the danger is that you can walk for miles in them, and get comfortable on your path. Why should we want to wear the Louboutin's? Who wants sore feet?

Lilly smiled to herself as she admired her new shoes on the shelf in her messy walk-in closet. She had never been a fan of flip flops, even at the beach, hers where usually rhinestone-studded with wedge heels. The new black Louboutin's were her gift to herself. She wrapped the soft cotton towel more snugly around her firm, but never quite slim enough, waist. Her newly highlighted hair was dripping down her face, damp from her shower. Today's luncheon had been a celebration of one of their most profitable years. And Lilly had been a monumental player in that milestone. After years of feeling a restlessness that gnawed at her mind, making her breathless with anxiety, she had finally found comfort in the mysterious question, who was she? When the jumble of thoughts in her mind had made her head pound like it was being hit with hail, out of control, untamable, she knew that if she didn't find something to focus on, she was spiraling to a place where darkness was comforting.

And so she had challenged herself, by getting more involved in the business she had long supported her husband in. She had always had her pinky in, but had she somehow known that someday it would be her redemption? She accomplished things she had done before, only better. She took on multiple tasks, completing them with that scary, overwhelming fear that could either freeze or energize. As her capabilities grew, her position was redefined in the minds of her husband and other business partners. Still Lilly demanded more of herself, needing to control her wandering mind. She accepted that this control was what she would need if she felt herself slipping towards the comforting darkness again. In this way, Lilly found herself. The more she conquered the more she found ways to push herself. It was with this growth, this confidence and stability that she found healing. Failing was never an option; she wasn't a quitter. This attitude, her fighting spirit, was what kept her from being attacked by the hungry, those that fed off the insecurities of the weak.

Lilly thought about the business, it was an accomplishment she was proud of, but her real happiness came from something much less financially profitable. Once her energy had been quieted, she began to live fearlessly in her personal life. She indulged her love of live music by going to listen to local bands, even if no one was available to join her, she forced herself to go alone. It got easier. She lived to try new things, sports, food, gyms, traveling to unique destinations. It was truly through this that she felt content.

Getting ready to have dinner with her long-time friends, Lilly turned to the mirror and started applying her make-up, looking at the straight blonde hair that defined structure and stability. In the foggy mirror she saw that hint of springy black. It would always be there. She smiled at her reflection and thought, who needed flip flops, when you could wear Louboutins?

They met at the same time, linking their arms around each other, seeing their faces from the past with the eyes of today. Sophia, with colors so true, so brilliant, they blinded those not open to accepting them. Ella, who's rainbow was attached to heaven by the silkiness of her heart. Lilly, the tigress, playing in the high, swaying grass, laughing at lurking danger. Flora, like wildflowers that bloom with the confidence of being. Together they reached for the doorbell.

She placed the last bottle on the table, because for tonight that would be enough. The lone bottle left on her Venice treasure was hers, but she would save that one. The five of them would sit around the table with the comfort of the years their hostess:

the entrepreneur, the artist, the spiritual, the courageous, and the writer; equally influential in the creation of the other. Called upon as needed, accommodating with their unique strengths. Each of them had started life the same, but different. Like the wines created in a vineyard. The pen, that was her mind, already immortalizing the scene in words.

They say vintage wines are the most enjoyable, that maturity allows them to fill our palette with an intoxicating burst of complex flavors. Some of these wines may have been created in prestigious, longstanding wineries, while others may have been born in the last desperate effort to overcome difficulties, or created during conflict and crisis. Even though they all lay there proudly, side by side, together... their different labels were just the introduction to the experience you would embark on when you choose to savor one. These women were truly like fine wine, they all have a journey that created their individuality, their complexity... and if you are lucky enough to sip from their beautiful souls, you will forever be enchanted. The doorbell rang, they were here she thought; my vintage collection.

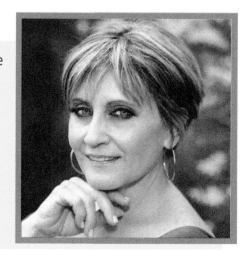

Lucia Colangelo has been writing since the day she picked up a crayon. She is currently writing the continuation of My Vintage Collection to be published Fall 2017, in the new Sisterhood ƒolios, Born To Be Me.
Lucia lives in Toronto with her family. When she's not writing she enjoys traveling, reading, gourmet pizza, pasta, lattes and wine.

Marla David

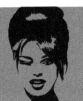

When I was around five years old, in a casual conversation, my mother informed me that I was adopted. At that time, of course, I didn't know what that meant exactly. I did know one thing though – being adopted made me different in some way.

As I grew up, some of the pieces of the puzzle began to fill in. I learned that I was born from another woman. I learned the story – my story. My adoptive mom's brother, Willy, the family doctor, delivered me at the Doctor's Hospital. She went on to describe how I was then adopted. When I was five days old I was handed to her by my birth mother, a Scottish woman. My birth mother was described as 'a little more filled out' than she was, with auburn colored, medium-length hair. She always finished the story with, "This all happened in front of Will's office on Dupont Street." I went through life with this short narrative, which impacted my life tremendously. This one great story of my life dictated how I lived my life, the choices I made, and was a part of me. It is said that your thoughts become your behaviors and, ultimately, your reality. This came true for me.

I believed I would adopt a child myself because I had been adopted. It seemed like the most natural thing because it was a story which I had rehearsed over and over through the years. Then, I always said I would travel to Scotland one day, to see if I felt some sort of connection to the land, and I did.

On my first solo trip when I was 40 years old, I went to England, Scotland and Wales. I considered it my heritage, having been naturally born to a Scottish woman. But I also had an identity problem. I didn't know where I belonged. I was between worlds. Not wanted in one, but not from the other. I know that seems, perhaps, a silly and unproductive way of thinking, but back then, it made perfect sense.

This by no means diminishes the love and respect I have always held for my parents. But I didn't know how they felt about me. I had to learn that.

This was not an easy task and I had a more difficult time picking up on some things. My family was not the most demonstrative when it came to expressing love. It doesn't mean it wasn't there, we just weren't the touchy-feely kind of family, especially when we got older. When I disappointed my parents, I felt that I lost their love. It was difficult to process. So, being adopted pushed my self-esteem down into the bottom of the well.

> Take it!
> Take another little piece of my heart now, baby,
> Oh, oh, break it!
> Break another little bit of my heart, now darling, yeah,

yeah, yeah, yeah,
Oh, oh, have a!
Have another little piece of my heart now, baby, hey,
You know you got it, child, if it makes you feel good
~Piece of My Heart, Janis Joplin

I also felt that my parents favored my sister because she was pretty and smart. I was an awkward kid; rather quiet and shy. People would find that hard to believe now, but it is true. I had a hard time 'fitting in', and I certainly was not part of the 'in group' at school, or at camp. Interestingly enough, even though I had my insecurities and low self-esteem, I was not unhappy. I really didn't know any different. This just felt like an adopted life.

I had my insular group of friends and my family while I was growing up. I was not a risk-taker, nor did I participate in anything other than what I had to. I was happy hanging around at home. Life was pretty predictable. Puberty and my teen years were extremely challenging at times because of my low self-esteem, but I managed to get through it. The clock did not stand still to wait for me to grow up emotionally or developmentally. One of my desires was that I wanted to be a mother, be a volunteer, and maybe even run the PTA at my kids' school. This was pretty far-fetched for a shy woman to believe, but it actually came to fruition, just like many of the stories I told myself. Every person has their own journey, and this has been mine. A lot of things I said I wanted to do, I have done. It's like I manifested my life right from the get-go.

I believed my stories – the ones other people said, or the ones I told myself. That little voice in my head continually played the recording so I wouldn't forget. My inner critic was my worst enemy, but then I learned how to shut it up, and use it to my benefit. These days the recording only plays things which support me. When I slip back to what was, I notice it, and correct that negative thought immediately. I have control over that part of me that wreaked havoc on my life for decades. Looking back I realize the stories that defined me throughout my early years were good stories. After all, in this world any outcome could be plausible, so this was a very reassuring factor for me, even though it has taken a long time for me to figure this out. This realization only came when I was ready, and with a lot of inner work. The many books I read on personal development contributed to teaching me to figure out the 'what', and the 'how' of my journey. Taking my life and laying it out in front of me like a timeline made for an interesting narrative in itself. It's my story. I am very proud of it. This is something that I couldn't say a decade ago. But today, I see things differently.

> Before the risin' sun, we fly
> So many roads to choose
> We'll start out walkin' and learn to run
> (And yes, we've just begun)
> ~We've Only Just Begun, The Carpenters

Our whole life is made up of stories. Some stories though, aren't in the timeline we've laid out for ourselves. Going through divorce is an example of that. I am presently going through a second one. All the fanfare of a roaring circus is at hand and I am the main event. Divorce always seems to send you into outer space. But there is one thing that I know; there is life after divorce, and you do land again. I try not to let my divorce define me in any way. I've moved on and have begun a new chapter. What is in the past is over and done with. Time has a way of changing things. Would I have ever thought when I divorced my first husband I would be friends with him today? Not in a million years. But I am, and happy about this for the family. There is no reason why we can't be friends. Since I tend to live a heart-centered life, I am not one to be judgmental. I accept what is. I am happy things have worked out this way. I think it is a clear sign of maturity when two people can move beyond differences, to acceptance and understanding.

> Just passing through
> And it's no sacrifice
> Just a simple word
> It's two hearts living
> In two separate worlds
> But it's no sacrifice
> ~Sacrifice, Elton John

When I looked at my life from this different perspective, a more objective one, with the bigger picture in mind, and with compassion, I saw the pattern and the purpose. When I factored faith into each story of my life, it gave the stories new meaning. Each one involved my heart in some way. So, that is why I say often that time helps, but it is love that ultimately heals. Time will help ease the pain and suffering, but until you factor in love, there isn't the final shift that takes you over the final peak to complete healing. Like riding the wave of ecstasy, it isn't until you go over the edge, and experience an orgasm, that you feel completed and satisfied. That is the added ingredient needed to hit it out of the ballpark.

With that said, I realize I am now unmasked - living a new story, a new chapter in my life. I have changed and my life now reflects those changes.

> "Life on this planet is an adventure – from the moment we're born until the time we take our last breath. Life is a madcap caper – scary, exhilarating, boring, peaceful, and loving. Life is a quest. Life is a thrill. Life is a romance. Life is a lark. Life is!"
> ~Louise Hay

I couldn't agree with her more. I see that life is there for me to knead and mold, as I would a piece of clay. This will enable me to bring out the magnificence which lays dormant in me.

If I don't grab the reins of my life, life will just happen to me. I would rather be in the driver's seat. There is so much I can do to influence my own existence - to enhance my story. Why should I not take life up on this opportunity?

> Too often, the opportunity knocks,
> But by the time you push back the chain,
> Push back the bolt, unhook the two locks
> And shut off the burglar alarm, it's too late.
> ~Rita Coolidge

I never know when opportunity knocks. Frankly, I don't even know if I would recognize an opportunity or even be ready for it if it was standing in my doorway. I don't have expectations that everything is handed to me in life on a silver platter, either. I believe that sometimes when I march to my own drummer, so to speak, I can take the road less traveled, and I may come across something far more interesting. But mostly in life, if I don't know about it, I don't know what I am missing. That is why I have to take the initiative. Nothing happened for me until I was prepared to take action. Just thinking things doesn't get the job done. Not until I was engaged was there some outcome.

Since I have learned that action is the secret ingredient to my success and the pursuing of my passions, I have honed my organizational skills, and set goals. I set immediate, interim and long-term goals, and I remember to reward myself each babystep of the way. I have resorted to making lists, and I remember to include on the list the things which have priority, the things I really could be doing, and the things I would like to do, but are not necessary. This has helped me tremendously. Since I have started this, I have accomplished so much.

> Stop waiting for creative inspiration. Start creating and inspire yourself along the way.
> ~ Ryan Lilly

I have noticed the next generation sees things differently. They tend to fear less when it comes to living life large. My three daughters constantly take action toward things which ignite their souls. They enjoy travel and the finer things in life, yet they have their feet planted firmly on the ground. I see that they are not afraid to step out of their comfort zone. They think 'outside the box' and take action toward their goals. I believe that when there is something that really scares you, this is where you need to go. As I do this more often, it becomes easier. Once I started stepping out the box more, I really began to grow. Personal development has become my ally and my lifeline.

Gratitude and forgiveness have both been integral in living a heart-centered life. I am grateful for the little things. I forgive others, and mostly myself, for everything. I do little things; tweak my reality in order to live my best life. It is always the little things which elicit change. It always starts with baby steps. I started to recite what I was grateful for each morning as I woke up and each evening as I lay in bed before I slept. I spent one year doing something each day to pay it forward, honoring the gratitude I felt in my heart. I continue to do so. It became important for me to just love, and be love; to feel love and embrace it, doing my best to allow my love to shine out. This is what healed me and brought me to where I am today.

I am blessed.

Since it is important to take the time each day to ignite my soul, I find myself doing those small things which give me joy. It is in the little things - little pieces of joy. I do my gratitude list, meditate, or do other things, too. I remember to practice self-care. This is important, because just like everyone else, I live a pretty hectic life most of the time. It is vital I recharge by getting off the treadmill in order to heal and just 'be'. This has brought a sense of peace in my life. This is part of my daily regimen, and I am so happy I have achieved this, as it has been such a huge part of my healing and growth.

> And to do what your heart's telling you
> I have found
> That to make life worth living
> You must have a dream
> Fit this of your own to pursue
> I may falter from time to time but then life
> Well, what would it mean
> If mountains were easy to climb?
> ~If Mountains Were Easy to Climb, Mrs. Henderson Presents

Looking back on my life thus far, I feel my greatest achievement is having the capacity to love. Having my three daughters, and now a granddaughter, showed me what love 'is'. How fortunate to have three healthy and beautiful daughters, each special in their own way. I succeeded in becoming a mother, despite the challenges thrown my way. Now I am a grandmother. How joyous! It is quite astonishing that I never had a desire to 'be' anything other than a mother. Accomplishing this has validated me immensely, and has given my life a special purpose. In hindsight, this equates to me being a success, by my standards. At this stage in my life, I don't care if society dictates success differently. I am content and my success has helped build self-confidence. It has helped me grow wings and develop as a person exponentially. I have my daughters to thank for that. I am very grateful for my dogs, who have taught me how to love unconditionally. They have always been there for me; they make me happy, light-spirited, and they make me laugh. I call them puppies, because dogs never really grow up. They stay in that cute and playful state most of their lives. This year I have lost some fur-babies, and it has been a heart-wrenching time for me. I think of them with love, knowing that they will always be with me in my memories, and my grief is lessened.

> If the sun refused to shine, I would still be loving you
> When mountains crumble to the sea, there will still be
> you and me.
> ~Thank You, Led Zeppelin

A new narrative I am now feeding myself is – that I am a success and I am self-confident. I am loved, lovable, and I love. I love life, and life loves me. Not all the time, of course, do things work out exactly as I would like. That is the way of the world. I cannot have the good without some bad. It sure makes me appreciate things in my life more. If there were no hurdles for me to jump over, life would be boring. But it is the challenges that I faced in my life that have proven to be the greatest learning opportunities. After I have had a bad turn, when I have something good, I relish it and cherish it with all my heart. Even if it is just a little thing, it doesn't matter. It is the little pieces which make up the whole; the pieces of my heart.

Aside from health, family, happiness, and comforts, the most important thing is peace of mind. It is through the little things, small pieces adding up, that create a sense of serenity and calm in my world. This sustains me through the harder times, when life challenges me. I love my pieces. Each piece contributes to my well-being. I try to add more pieces all the time – new pieces which come from living a heart-centered life; expressing my love in little ways, and often. That is what ignites my soul and allows me to live life large. Home isn't in Scotland or anywhere else. Home resides right inside of me in my heart-center. They are totally correct when they say that home is where your heart is. It is where I have planted roots, the foundation where I'm at peace, and connection to memories that are who I am, such as family and raising my children.

As I continue to turn more pages of my life, my purpose gets clearer. I find an ease which I think is attributed to the many ways I stretch myself and grow. When I read, I learn. It is clear to me that I need to pursue my passions. Life is too short to not do what you love, and enjoy life as best you can. I am not here just to survive. I want to thrive. By pursuing my passions, I feel balanced and peaceful. My passions are kind of like muses which help me align with my soul.

Writing is like a muse. The 'art of the story' started way back when cavemen would act out their story to their tribe. After all - storytelling is about life. Thoughts and words are in me, and I am just letting them out, just as Michelangelo carved the sculpture from the stone by merely taking away the excess; the sculpture was inside all along. When my words convey a message, they have planted a seed which creates a ripple effect. This has the power to make changes or create a shift in another's life in a positive way. This is a very powerful and useful tool. It is extremely gratifying to have people express this to me in person. It is very humbling. Through the art of writing, I have found my voice. By honoring the call to write, I feel I am celebrating my true path in this lifetime. I am leaving a legacy because it is not as much what you do for others, as it is what you instill in them – adding value that will carry on inside of them. It constantly takes me out of my comfort zone, but is also therapeutic and cathartic. I am putting in writing my journey of self-exploration. By putting it down on paper, it puts my life into perspective. Writing has given my life new purpose, and has brought me to where I am today, an international bestselling author. I am grateful, and humbled.

> If you do not breathe through writing, if you do not cry out in writing, or sing in writing, then don't write, because our culture has no use for it.
> ~Anais Nin

There is a concept in Taoism called Wu wei. This is when you are doing nothing, just being in a calm state allowing things to happen naturally the way they are supposed to. I try hard to live a heart-centered life. Meditation has helped me quiet my mind and just 'be' as in Wu wei. In the madness of this world, meditation takes the circus out of my brain and allows it to rest, which then allows my body and soul to follow suit. Meditation has taught me that all that matters right now in this space and time is the breath in this very moment. As I meditate, my body, mind and spirit come together to nurture me. Laughing and smiling are also therapeutic for me. I do things which I love and this makes me content. Living my life of passion has become 'the way' for me. I need to do the things which make me come alive, such as listening to music. The music and lyrics, like a really good book, transport me to another place. It goes without saying that joy comes from being with my family and friends. I could say the same about being with my dogs, and then – there is my garden.

> Be like a flower and turn your face to the sun.
> ~Kahlil Gibran

As a nature lover, and a nature momma, I take my garden seriously. Sinking my hands in the soil, weeding, pruning, even planting, I try to make it a habitat which is complementary to nature in every sense. When I commune with nature, I am swathed in good feelings. It is like taking a vitamin pill for my soul. My garden is something I enjoy working on and spending time in. It is my oasis and retreat. The rewards beyond the soul-feeding are the abundance of birds, butterflies, and other wild species that visit my garden. That validates my efforts, bringing me more joy by contributing positively to the environment and wildlife. As I tend to my garden, I also have been cultivating my life garden, planting seeds and harvesting as the years go by. I know it is important to give in life, in order to get. That is why I live my life of passion, now. I have found my passions and live each day focusing on them to the best of my ability. I am designing my own future and creating my heaven on earth, in alignment to the beating of my heart's desire.

> We can never know about the days to come
> But we think about them anyway, yay
> ~Anticipation, Carole King

I anticipate great things in the future. I am fascinated by the mystery of what could be because I embrace the belief that there are limitless possibilities out there. There is so much happening and I know more great things will come. I am exhilarated thinking about this. That is why I need so badly to continue to grow as a person, and as a soul. I need to follow my passions and through them, I will continue on my path toward my destiny.

I had to learn to love and be kinder to myself. It's like I finally learned self-respect. After all, how could I possibly expect others to respect me if I didn't respect myself first? I do mirror work, where I stand in front of the mirror and say positive things about myself, to myself. I tell myself I am fabulous, beautiful, loved and smart, for example. I believe in the Golden Rule – Do unto others, as you would have them do unto you.

I try to experience every emotion possible as I am living my story. I consider myself an empath. I feel for people and situations. I often don't like being in this game of Life. I can be afraid and try to protect myself from people, or things, criticism, or harsh realities. I can hide, but then I may miss the wonderful adventure that's available for me.

Everyone is afraid of something, but I know I can do it anyway. I have already proven that. I have rewritten the script of my life.

> It's a new horizon and I'm awakin' now
> Oh I see myself in a brand new way
> The sun is shinin'
> ~Don't Look Back, Boston

Changing my thoughts changed my paradigm. All those stories I fed myself that helped make me who I was, have now morphed as I have done an auto-correct to clean out the snags which hampered my growth and stopped me from pursuing my destiny. This new thinking created a different paradigm, and I initiated new actions which serve me better. It has been a long process to learn, and there is still many steps on my path. I have become a sponge for learning in this life classroom. It has allowed me to grow, confront my fears and insecurities, and led me to where I am today. Being open to new adventures has breathed new life into me; almost like having a transfusion. I am taking the road less traveled, walking directly toward uncharted territory, and perhaps, even more challenges. I believe that this way of thinking, although it may bring more adversity, will also provide me with a richer and more fulfilling life.

Writing a new narrative has aligned with my authentic self – the Marla I have grown back into; the pure soul I was at birth, I am again. A good story doesn't have to begin with 'Once Upon a Time' or end with 'Happily Ever After'. We live in an imperfect world. It just has to be a good story. I told myself stories right from the start. With examination of my experiences, I make edits to my life script whenever

I feel the need to create something else which will work for me better, and which brings me more happiness and love. I tweak my life in order to live my best life. I love that I have the ability and freedom of choice to do that. I enjoy being flexible to change, as I am an ever-evolving person. As change is a certainty in life, acceptance helps me be more resilient. I have grown stronger through this process. As I surrender to the rhythm of life, I am confident that as I finish each chapter, I will let the light shine from within me, and there will be many new and wonderful stories to write and live out.

> But the fact is, she [the muse] won't be summoned. She alights when it damn well pleases her. She falls in love with one artist, then desert him for another. She's a real bitch!
> ~Erica Jong, Seducing the Demon: Writing for My Life

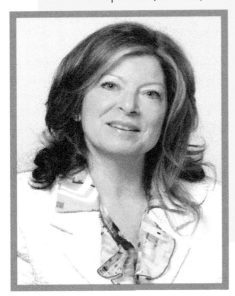

Marla David is a Life Coach (Positive Lifestyle Coaching), speaker, writer, co-author of four #1 International Bestsellers (Empowering Women to Succeed Volume II: From Burnout to Victory, 365 Moments of Grace, 365 Life Shifts & Empowering Women to Succeed Volume III: Bounce). A retired stay-at-home mom of three grown daughters, and a granddaughter, Marla lives her life of passion each day, spending time with family and friends, her dogs, and enjoying travel, nature, arts, and culture.

Lauren Dickson

On the Wrong Side of Love

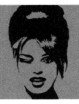

Holding on, and letting go. Two polar opposites, but they both can be so excruciatingly hard and painful. Holding on, when you should let go, will ultimately hurt you much more. There was a frustration and an emptiness that permeated my heart and lungs, and limited my ability to think and even breathe because I needed to let go. Sometimes I hate how much I feel. I hate how 'they' never realize how much love, compassion, and effort I put in. I hate that I can't make it as painfully obvious as it is in the abyss of my heart; as deeply and forcefully it takes over every fiber of my being.

Growing up I never had a 'Daddy's little girl' type of relationship with my father. He was never one to open up or express his feelings; perhaps he wasn't sure how. My parents fought often while I was growing up, which eventually lead to their separation in 1997. Also, my eldest brother was verbally abusive, and otherwise rough with me growing up; it is only in our adult years that we get along better. So needless to say, I did not have good male connections while growing up. On top of a stressful home situation I was bullied at school. These were all contributing factors with some depression and anxiety beginning in my teen years. Despite that stress, I managed to remain empathetic and considerate toward others. In witnessing what I grew up, with I told myself that when the time came for love I would not make the same mistakes they did in their relationship. On the journey towards love finding me, however, I dealt with a tumultuous string of men who never actually gave a crap about me. They only cared about their terms, needs, timing, and wants.

I honestly don't think I have ever been truly loved by a single hand that has touched me. When I started dating my first boyfriend in 2010, at the age of 21 it was a thrilling time. Not only my first serious dating experience, but that a guy five years older than me was actually interested. To be desired, cared for, and to have your heart awakened is probably a wish we all long to come true. It wasn't until after that relationship had ended that I figured out I needed to know and love myself more first before I could ever truly love or be loved in return. He claimed early on that he loved me, but it wasn't until after the relationship ended, that I realized that he never really loved me; he was only 'in love' with the idea of me. The night it ended I was left at midnight out in the pouring rain, and for some time after that my heart felt as though it was still stuck out in the dark, and in the rain. To this day he is the only guy that has ever claimed he loved me, and yet it wasn't even real love. He had an idea in his head of how he wanted the relationship to go. He wanted me to move in with him way too soon, and I'm so glad I didn't. He had anger issues, and when the milestones of the relationship were not going according to his short timeline, he freaked out, and ended it. I was devastated. I felt abandoned. This man, who was talking about our future, and our future children, had completely given up on me at the first sign of a bump in the road. I had given my heart and body to this man that I loved, and supported him emotionally while he was still building his own life. He was selfish and angry that I was not yet at the place he thought I should have been at in my life.

I had fallen back into a bit of a depression following that. I felt stuck in a rut of letting that pain take over my every breath and thought. The stress took a toll on my already petite frame and I lost some weight, but also lost the small sense of self-esteem I had at the time. After the initial devastation and heartache, and what felt like constant tears of pain and loss, I realized that it was a blessing in disguise. That relationship, and the demise of that relationship, was actually the start of me getting my life back on track. He never truly loved me, but at the time, I don't think I truly loved myself. It was then that I began a long journey of self-discovery, soul searching, and living my purpose.

It was over a year before I could bring myself to attempt to date again. At the advice of friends I reluctantly began online dating. I was very skeptical about it, but thought I would give it a try. So help me God, I will never go back to online dating, as nothing good came from it for me. It was nothing but a string of men who would try to tell me what they thought I wanted to hear, just to try to get me into bed. Guys who would only call me when they were not seeing anyone else; or late nights when they were lonely. Guys who I found out were seeing someone else, but still wanted to keep me on the side. I had built up some backbone from my first relationship, but still somehow found myself falling into the pathetic trap of men having their way with me. I hate to admit it, but I think I just craved any attention I could get from a guy.

That isn't really me at all, so for a time I beat myself up over it; pretending those guys actually cared about me just to serve some insecurity in myself. Some of them I even gave multiple chances. Why? Looking back I am shaking my head at my own behavior.

I eventually stood up more for myself; called them out on their bull, and ignored the guys who would weeks - or even months later, try to contact me. I think God was testing me to see if I would have the self-respect to not even acknowledge their attempt, and I did just that. I no longer let the negative energy seep through. I sometimes would ask God why he would keep bringing these bad guys into my life. It wasn't so much heartbreaking or painful dealing with the 'bad guys'; it was more frustrating and stressful. I knew they were bad for me, so I was not losing something from my life. It was all making me stronger. It was helping build my self-respect, my self-worth, and knowing I deserved a heck of a lot better! Keep in mind, none of these guys were ever officially my boyfriend, other than my first boyfriend from 2010. Ironically enough, the only official relationship I have had was at a time when I was not ready, or grown enough into my individual self. Yet in the years since, I have come to know myself in the deepest of ways; in my heart and soul, and have become more prepared to let love come find me when it is time.

The last guy I dated from the online dating world was a guy who had actually shown that he cared for me. We were comfortable with each other. He was showing a lot of interest and excitement towards me. Unlike other guys from my past experience, he had his life together;

good job, a house of his own. When our brief tango ended, he claimed it was due to his anxiety, which I knew he had (something we had in common). He said he thought he was ready, but wasn't. I was speechless at first. I was not in a hurry for a relationship. I just wanted to continue on the path we were on and continue getting to know each other. He thought it was best to just cut the cord. I began to over-analyze every detail of our relationship trying to figure out where things had gone wrong. It just didn't make sense.

As much as I feel so very deeply with my heart and soul, I also have been in my head way too much. That is something I have improved upon immensely. My mind was trying to make sense of it all; running conversation scenarios through my mind like a song on repeat of all the things I wish I had said, but didn't. Hindsight is a funny thing. There was an awful, paralyzing feeling of knowing there was nothing I could do. I could not convince him to stay if he was hell-bent on leaving.

It was after that I just wanted to shut off emotionally. I did not want to try anymore. I felt as though all of my effort and care was going to waste, and not being reciprocated. As much as I love seeing others happily in love, I became almost sick of seeing happy couples. It's not that I feel I need man to be happy. I am independent, and I create my own happiness. It's just that on this journey of this often unfair, harsh world, love can be that one blindingly beautiful presence that makes life so much more fulfilling. I felt like I had reached that exact point which I had prayed so hard to keep me from.

That point was fear; fear of trusting a man again. I didn't want to be that woman with 'trust issues,' but I was not the one who was not letting someone in. It was others who pushed me away; wanted a convenient relationship instead of a commitment. There were times where the emotional pain left an actual physical pain in my heart. There were moments where I would bawl my eyes out and feel like I could cry forever. Then there were other times where I felt like I had no tears left to cry. I had reached a point where I had adapted and transformed to be resilient. As much as the pain was at times overwhelming, I did not let it keep me down.

In the times between each guy that stormed in and out of my life, I found more of myself. I learned more; what I deserved, what I needed and wanted in a partner; I progressed further in my personal development of loving every bit of myself first. I fell in love with myself, and my life - every bright, bubbly piece, and every dark corner to the deepest depths of my true being. I welcome and make time for the passions and opportunities that light a fire within me. The hope of a spark that triggers rapture within, and fills your heart with so much love and energy, you feel like you could soar into the sky and fly! This is the real me!

They say things happen when you least expect it. I stopped dating for a bit, and just focused on making my own life as beautiful as I want it to be. One of the many things I love about myself is that I never let all the crap, pain, and heartache keep me down. I always pick myself back up again, and keep pushing forward. My most recent surprise is that I met someone the old-fashioned way - completely out of the blue. God clearly wanted me to meet this man because chance encounters are rare in the busy industry I work in.

It was like a breath of fresh air. A man unlike anyone else I had ever met. There was just something about him. Sometimes just knowing there's something different says it all; that even the most eloquent words don't even do it justice. There was chemistry, and an intellectual connection. I had real conversations with him, and although neither of us wanted to rush into a relationship, that made me more physically attracted to him; his natural rugged looks were enhanced by his energy, zest, and passion for life. A few weeks in I found myself to be the one holding the conversations, and initiating plans; the vibe was different. I was enjoying our developing relationship and wanted to wait for him to say what was on his mind. It was another few weeks before he simply said it wasn't going to work. In that moment I felt my heart sink, and a lonely ache overwhelmed my chest and stomach. I thought, "Oh here we go again!" I asked him why he didn't bring it up before, when he was first having doubts. He said he wanted to wait until he was sure, and that irked me. Sure of what? We had barely just begun, and there was so much more to explore about each other.

Here he was so sure of ending it, when I was sure there was potential. Ironically enough, in that moment of him letting me go, he was actually being more vulnerable with me, explaining heartbreak and betrayal from his past. It was sweet vulnerability, which was a beautiful spot to build from, not to end things on. He had a gentleness about him in that conversation I had never received from a man before, and that made it harder for me to let go. I saw in him the insecurities he has due to previous betrayal. I was angry and hurt for the initial way he handled it, but then, as comforting as that gentle sensitivity was, it actually hurt me even more. I wanted to experience his full heart, but he could not share. Once someone has their mind made up, no words or tears are going to change their mind, and the last thing I wanted was to beg him to give us a chance. I wanted him to respect the way I handled the heartbreak.

Too many people these days are too quick to rush sex, but the minute they could be getting closer to someone they bail and run for the hills, looking for 'the next best thing.' The best person for your life can often be the very one you're not giving a chance. He gave me a glimpse into his beautiful mind, heart, and soul, and left me wanting to know him more. One of the worst feelings is feeling unwanted by the person you may want the most. The longing is still there when I run into him from time to time. That's a new experience because with the previous men in my life, once they were gone, they were gone! We have slowly become friends, and it's good to have him in my life even in that way.

God had been removing people from my life that were not good for me. Even ones whom I thought were friends had shown their true colors; so-called friends whom I rarely, if ever, heard from unless I reached out to them. I stopped reaching out. No true friend is ever that busy that they can't send a quick text to see how you are, or God forbid people still made phone calls these days! I am very busy, but I always make time for the people that I consider important to me. It's all about priorities and who you make time for. I was angry at God over this, and I think He was okay with that. He finally brought someone into my life who matched my energy and passion for life, and then he ripped him away, or so I thought. I remember falling down the stairs, sustaining bruising on my arm and bottom. Looking at those bruises in the mirror, I began to cry; not for any physical pain, but for the reminder of the emotional bruises on my heart and the draining bruises on my mind from overthinking every last detail of why things happened the way they did.

I don't define my life based on who is in it or not, but I do long to have a deep, everlasting connection with someone. I think that ultimately the big lesson with the anguish over the years from those who used, abused, and cheated me, and even from this budding romance turned friendship, is that I have come to appreciate myself more. I have come to not only appreciate, but thoroughly enjoy solitude. I have awakened my own soul, instead of waiting for someone to come along and do it for me. I see people who don't know who they are without their partner. They define their own identity by the presence or absence of another. I've seen people dwell on a breakup, only to blindly jump into another relationship without giving themselves the much needed time and space to learn from that past experience. I have learned to make myself whole first. I don't want to find my 'other half.' I want to find a soul who is already whole to combine with my whole heart and soul as well. I have had to pick up the pieces of my own crushed heart, and made art with the pieces.

Perhaps this most recent man in my life is not meant to be the one for me; but he has shown me examples of the qualities I wish to have in a forever partner. Those amazingly deep craters of substance captivated my soul, and allowed me to release my wilder, more liberated side that I had somewhat hidden in the shadows of my shaken soul. I sometimes wish he would have waited long enough to see every side of me. I am like a book that you will never quite finish; every beat and passion within me is a new page waiting to be turned and discovered. In a way, it is sad that I have yet to meet someone who yearns to dive into the depths of my soul and unwrap my every thought, dream, fear, and ambition. On the other hand, I feel empowered that I have so much to offer. There is power in knowing I still have yet to be truly and fully discovered by the right one. The one who wants to become so intimately attached to all of the in-between bits of me, and all of the gory, savage bits of me, all while opening up all of their gorgeous, gory bits too. I don't hate the falling hard; I hate the falling hard for those who did not deserve my love, my patience, and my understanding. Will there be more days ahead of heartache and pain? Well this is life, so yes... but I have more recently released the firm grasp and can feel a liberating sense of peace, knowing that who is meant to stay will stay, and who is meant to go will go. For every one who leaves, God has someone even greater in store for me, and I keep my hope in that.

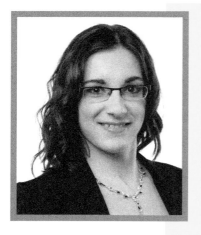

Lauren Dickson is an all-around creative, old soul and certified wedding coordinator, as well as being the Associate Manager of Events & Logistics for Canada Fashion Group. Through her own struggles and heartache, she has built self-resiliency and a deeper connection and love for herself. It is through her own experiences and compassionate demeanor that she hopes to impact and inspire others to fight their demons, discover their authentic individuality, and fully embrace life, not just survive it.

Jennifer Febel

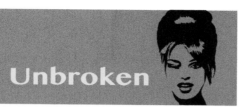

Unbroken

I was nineteen when I received my official diagnosis, but of course by then I had already been suffering in silence for years. Anorexia. Bulimia. Major Depression. Generalized Anxiety. Obsessive Compulsive Disorder. Suicidal ideation. And self-harm (which means there are scars on my body that I put there).

In other words: broken.

Every doctor I saw, every specialist I consulted all agreed; I was broken. And they were right, because when you're told over and over again by very smart people with lots of letters after their names that you are broken, well... eventually you begin to believe them.

I wasn't born broken.

In fact, according to the great Aristotle, one of my favorite philosophers (yes, I have a favorite philosopher because I'm nerdy like that), we are born perfect; blank slates upon which life inscribes her Journey. Tabula Rasa, which literally means "blank slate" means that no one is born broken so,

I could not have been born broken, no one could. Even if it doesn't always feel that way. Growing up I didn't feel broken.

In fact, I had what I considered to be a very normal upbringing and spent my childhood doing the usual childhood things. I had plenty of friends, I did well in school and I had the usual childhood experiences including first crushes, chickenpox, dance classes, and sleepovers. And yet, as time went on the pain got worse, the fear got bigger, and my body began to crack under the pressure.

My earliest memories are of hospitals. When I was two years old I was diagnosed with a rare kind of heart murmur, the kind that makes even doctors scratch their heads and ask, "What is PDA?" Patent Ductus Arteriosus is a benign condition in which one of the arteries near the heart remains open after birth allowing blood and vital oxygen to bypass the lungs. Nowadays, this can be easily corrected with day surgery, but back in the early 1980's, this type of murmur was rare, and the surgery to correct it had only been performed a handful of times in Canada. Because the murmur was so loud, the doctors were having a hard time deciding if it was just PDA, or if there was a defect inside the heart as well. Consequently, I spent weeks in the hospital, both before and after my surgery, undergoing tests and scans and, finally, a nine-hour surgery and recovery. You would expect that I would have been upset being away from home, away from my family. But I loved it. I loved the attention; I loved the quiet. I loved having my own TV that I could watch, and my own dinner that was just for me. Being so young you would think I wouldn't remember any of it, but I do. I remember more than most.

From a very young age I also remember hating myself. Fast forward a bit and I'm five years old, playing in my room, and I remember digging my fingernails into my thigh; punishing myself for doing something wrong and knowing, with certainty, that I deserved it. The pain was still quiet; still easy to avoid, but the pressure was building.

I've often wondered, over the years, where such intense self-loathing came from. Where does a five-year-old learn to hate herself so much that she feels the need to cause herself physical pain? In examining this question I have had to face some hard truths about my childhood. Truths that, to this day, I am still attempting to reconcile.

From the outside, my family was loving and supportive; a little nuts, perhaps, but always there for each other. Or so I thought. It's amazing what you can find hidden in the shadows, and, unfortunately, the closer I looked the more I could see. While outwardly everything was wonderful, behind closed doors a different story emerged. A sister who couldn't love me. A mother who put her own needs first. Words portrayed as soothing caused scars deeper than you can imagine, and, just because they are invisible, make no mistake, they can still bleed.

Things really began to get bad as I neared my final days of high school. From the outside, everything seemed great! My GPA was 4.0, I had my pick of universities, and an incredible circle of friends. I find myself appreciating and loving these relationships more and more, the older I get. I think they saved me, actually, even if they don't know it. But no matter what I did, or how successful I was, the pain got worse and the fear got bigger.

Have you ever felt something wasn't right but you couldn't quite put your finger on it? In astronomy there's actually a name for this (hey, I told you I was a nerd). Averted vision is a well-known scientific phenomenon that states, when viewing fainter stars with the naked eye you need to look just to the side rather than directly at the star in order to really see it. Biologically, this is because of the disbursement of light-detecting cells in the retina of our eyes. And like a shadow seen only out of the corner of your eye, I, too, found the harder I tried to look at the cause of my pain, the less I was able to see.

And so I began to break.

The first time I began to notice the cracks was right before my high school prom. It's so cliché isn't it? And I hate that I'm a cliché, but I really did want to transform myself that night and have everyone notice me. Notice me and say, "Wow, look how beautiful she is." It was one week away from prom and my mom and I were at the dress shop for a final fitting to ensure the alterations were done correctly. I was in love with my dress. I had picked out a beautiful, soft yellow, chiffon gown, and I was so excited to wear it. But when I went to try it on we found it was a little snugger than it was supposed to be – they had taken it in too much. And instead of saying, "Oh, nuts, they botched the alteration," my mom asked me instead, "Did you gain weight?" And in that moment, something snapped inside me. It was an innocent enough comment, but like the straw that broke the camel's back, in that moment, I decided that I would fit into that dress. No. Matter. What. And in making that decision I stepped through the looking glass and into the world of eating disorders.

That summer I starved myself down over 40 pounds existing on a diet of pills and a mere 300 calories a day. My own friends barely recognized me. And still the pain got deeper and the fear got bigger.

People tend to think eating disorders are just about weight, or getting attention. This certainly plays a part, but consider this: an anorexic uses their conscious will power to override their body's own built-in self-preservation mechanism. It is a slow suicide; death by a thousand paper cuts.

It is about fear and control. It is about self-loathing and shame.

Anorexia is born of a profound and persistent desire to destroy and obliterate the Self, to literally disappear from existence. Trust me when I tell you, that the level of pain and shame that is required to literally starve yourself to death is not the result of not having a flat tummy or wanting to be a size 2. It comes from a much deeper, much darker place. I know. I've been there.

I've always been what you would call an over-achiever. I am the one who is always prepared, always organized, and always growing. In high school I was on the honor roll; in university I was top of my class. Whatever I do, I do it well, and I put my heart and soul into it. Which is what made my eating disorder all the more devastating. But it wasn't until I got my 'official diagnosis' that I really thought I was broken.

I remember sitting with my mom in the waiting room of a prominent psychologist in the suburbs of Toronto that summer. The walls were a god-awful shade of pink;

the kind of pink usually reserved for nursing home carpets, or funeral homes. I was scared. After months of vicious anxiety, crushing sadness, and the loss of a significant amount of weight, I knew something was wrong but I just couldn't figure out why I couldn't stop. My arms bore the scars of my pain, deep cuts made by my own hand in an attempt to reconcile the depths of agony I was experiencing. I remember asking myself often, "Am I crazy? I must be crazy. But do crazy people question their sanity? In which case the fact that I'm asking if I'm crazy must mean that I'm not crazy." I would play these questions over and over in my mind. I remember hoping that the doctor would recommend I be admitted to the psych ward because all I wanted was for the pain to end. The only way I could think that could ever happen was if I was medicated into a stupor. Upon hearing the diagnosis my mom was furious, and I never went back to that horrid pink office again. But the diagnosis followed me out the door.

Through all of it, I still managed to graduate high school with honors, attend university, and make the Dean's list. But with each passing day, the pressure continued to build; the pain became unbearable and the fear consumed me.

I finally broke.

The day started off surprisingly well. I was feeling good. I had seen my therapist earlier that day and things were going quite nicely, all things considered. After months and months of adjusting my medication we had finally found a mix that was working and didn't send me into a manic state. I hadn't hurt myself in nearly a week, which was a new record, and I had systematically gone through, and come clean about all my stashes of sharp objects. I had thrown

84

them all away, removing all temptation; something my therapist had recommended. It was the weekend and I was in my first year of university and working on a research project for my philosophy class. I remember that I had gone looking for a paperclip, which always ended up at the bottom of my drawer. And as I was looking and moving things around in the drawer I noticed something sharp that I had not yet disposed of, and so I gave it to my parents to throw away. And then I lost... My... Shit.

Suddenly the reality of my situation came crashing down on me – I had nothing left to hurt myself with, and the thought of that sent me spiraling into a breakdown of epic proportions. I was hysterical and I couldn't get control back. Have you ever seen the scene in Grays Anatomy where Cristina breaks down and can't stop crying? It was like that – only it wasn't happening to a character in a show. It was happening to me. My parents tried frantically to calm me down but nothing was working. No matter what I did I just couldn't stop shaking. I couldn't stop crying. That's when we decided it was time for me to go to the hospital.

I remember very little about the rest of that night. Memories come to me in flashes; little snippets of a movie that I know I've seen but the details are a blur. I remember sitting under one of those old TVs they used to have screwed into a corner on the wall (these were the days before flat screens) and I remember wishing it would fall on me so the pain would stop.

I remember meeting with the on-call psychologist, a weenie little guy with a receding hairline and a bowtie (a frickin' bow tie!).

I remember the scratchy feel of the hospital gown against my body and how I kind of liked it and found it comforting.

I remember my dad going out to a local donut shop at 3:00 a.m. and bringing back a batch of fresh-from-the-oven cheddar biscuits.

And I remember Dwayne, an incredible soul who was part of the hospital's Crisis Team (a team I would meet many more times over the coming years). He was the first person to acknowledge me. To notice me, not just my pain. And he was the first person who told me I was not broken. It would take me another 13 years of pain and darkness and fighting to finally understand his message.

In Japan, there exists a beautiful art form known as Kintsukuroi (keen-tsoo-koo-roy), which means literally 'to repair with gold'. It is the art of repairing pottery with molten gold or silver, in essence highlighting the scars of the break. Rather than attempt to hide the injury or pretend it never happened, the Japanese understand that the piece is more beautiful for having been broken and healed.

You see, life is a process of change and re-birth. The old systems and ways break down to make way for new learnings and realizations. It is beautiful and painful and poetic. It is simultaneously wonderful and horrible.

Change is inevitable, and yet we hold on to the old ways so tight that it is not the change itself that hurts, only our reluctance to embrace a new way. I never really understood the idea of surrendering, but after drowning in my pain for over a decade it became very clear. Learning to surrender is about learning to let go even when every fiber in your being wants to cling tight. Letting go is harder, but it will hurt less once you surrender.

No one is ever broken because we were never whole to begin with. We are in a constant state of change, of breaking down and building back up. Each time learning more. Each time becoming stronger. A broken bone is known to heal stronger than before the injury. A broken limb will never lose the scar of its journey but it is stronger for having healed, and can never break the same way again. It is unbroken.

Just as our bones break and heal stronger, so, too, do our minds. And so the goal is not to be whole, for that is just an illusion. Aim, instead to be stronger. Wiser. Unbroken.

It has been six years since I walked away from my eating disorder and began my journey back to health. Like all big decisions, this, too, came as an epiphany. It was a definite decision that took me down to the darkness, and a decision that brought me back out. The power of our decisions is astounding. In a split second – BAM! – you can decide to do something different and completely change your reality. And while we all have this ability all of the time, it is typically only during periods of extreme turmoil that we actually choose to tune in to this ability and change our lives.

My moment of clarity came a year after losing my father to liver disease. In the wake of my grief, my eating disorder had worsened. I spent my days planning my binges, and then purging everything I had eaten. I was in constant pain and I knew that I couldn't continue on. So I made a decision. I knew what would happen if I continued on the same path. I had already lost several friends to eating disorders and, regardless of what society thinks, those of us who suffer from anorexia or bulimia are acutely aware of the damage we are doing to our bodies. I knew that if I continued at that pace, it was only a matter of time before my body gave out. And so I decided to choose a different pain, the pain of recovery. Because even though it was equally as painful (if not, more so), at least it was a pain fueled by hope. And so back out of the looking glass I went.

The only way out is through. This was my mantra and this is what I clung to as I moved through the pain of recovery (and make no mistake – recovering from an eating disorder is incredibly painful - physically and emotionally). After years of denying my body nourishment I had to learn again how to eat, how to notice my hunger and how to take care of myself. It has been a hard road and yet, it has not been as hard as I thought. Because once you make the decision to change, everything after that is just details.

Today, I am fully recovered, medication free, and thriving. I am blessed to have met and married my best friend, Brian, and his love and support these past 13 years have meant more to me than any words could ever express. In 2014 I made the decision to start my own business and am now honored to help guide others on their path to recovery, using the tools that helped me to help them heal through the pain of depression, anxiety and childhood trauma. Every client who finds their way to me brings me new learnings as well, and helps me heal at deeper levels. I am so grateful to all the amazing souls I have met on this Journey.

Live Life Unbroken. It's just three little words, but they have had such a profound impact on my life.

I hear so many people say that they are broken; that their problems are insurmountable. That they cannot be fixed. It hurts when I hear this, not just because it is awful to see a beautiful soul in pain, but because I have been there. And my message of hope remains: No one is ever broken.

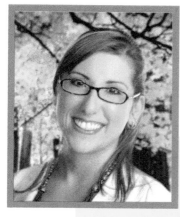

Jennifer Febel
Master Hypnotherapist, Wellness Coach,
Transformative Speaker

"You are not broken." This has become Jennifer's personal and professional mantra and it is one that she intends to spread to as many people as she can. As a Master Hypnotherapist, Coach, Trainer and Transformative Speaker, Jennifer helps free her clients from the distress of anxiety, depression and past trauma so they can find their inner peace and heal.

Andrea Judit

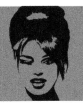

Unchained –
or I Was Married to a
Narcissist and Survived

"Be who you are and say what you feel, because those who mind don't matter and those who matter don't mind."
~Theodor S. Geisel aka Dr. Seuss

4:00 a.m. the light goes on. I was in a deep sleep. He starts yelling at me. I'm barely awake and I'm not sure of what is happening. Oh, he is really upset, yelling at me, getting up from bed and accusing me and my daughter and my mother that they don't accept him and they don't make him feel part of the family.

"Calm down – I love you, I accept you."

I'm trying to calm him down as usual. I just want to go back to sleep. The truth is that he was never really nice to them. When he went for dinner, he always criticized everybody, made the atmosphere stressed and very uncomfortable. No, they were not in love with him, but really there was no reason to be. He would always brag about himself but was not there to help them, or anyone. He only respected people with power: like the bank manager, the doctor and other people in key positions. He would be the most charming with them; kiss the ladies' hands. As it turned out, it is also a smart move of his manipulation process. But, what can I expect from someone who has no relationship with his own kids. I know he loves them, but he wants to manipulate them and he never really supports them or helps them or forgives them.

I grew up in Hungary. We were taught that family matters are important and family members want the very best for each other. My father was the main breadwinner. He had given everything he made to my mother. They were a tag team. Sometimes he had three jobs just to make our lives better. He really cared about and loved his family. I thought everyone was the same. How wrong I was!

When my first husband lost his job he was chasing a dream. It didn't even occur to him to go out and find another job to support his family. He expected to be supported by his family. It was so tough to be dependent on his family, to not be independent. I have always made my own money, worked and pursued my dream. I was actually driven by Spirit to do healing. First it came in as massage in the 1980's. I was told "nobody will want to be touched by you as your hands sweat." When I was anxious my hands would sweat. In spite of this, I was successful, giving the best massages to my clients.

I grew up being dependent on my family too. Finally, now, at the age of 57, I'm claiming my independence, through circumstances that are not so nice. "I want to be the person I want to be with."

I had never before seen a husband who doesn't want to help his wife but instead makes her look incompetent, puts her down, calls her fat. Who, when his wife needs help, tries to do the absolute minimum, making sure that she waited or was stressed enough just to make him feel better. Somehow this made him feel bigger, more powerful. What made me laugh, was when he complained about me to my family or friends. They felt really uncomfortable and didn't want to meet us again. These people knew me, loved me, respected me and didn't want to be subjected to such abuse.

I tried to make peace with his kids, but they never forgave me and blamed me because their parent's marriage had failed. I was a good scapegoat to hate - this way they didn't have to hate their own father. They didn't know that their parent's marriage had failed because it was not a healthy relationship.

I just happened to be there in the background.

Oh, we were so much in love. He noticed me, he paid attention to me. He really saw who I was and what I wanted and needed. I felt like I was in heaven.

"Don't mistake attention for respect."

My first husband was a passive aggressive, who didn't notice anything. I felt unseen, unappreciated, invisible in his eyes. So finally I am noticed. He must really love me. I didn't know it was just another manipulative technique - a sweet honeymoon to get to know, me really well so that later on, he can use it against me. He can intimidate me. He threw my precious books and my healing devices out in the garbage.

Oh, I'm a healer; I'm a holistic therapist, a doctor of natural medicine and an empath. I have spent the last 33 years learning to be the best in my profession. I love to read and I love to work on myself to grow better than I was, and learn new techniques to help others in a more efficient way. It is very beneficial to be a highly sensitive person when you do healing and have to feel the other person emotionally and physically. I can easily verify what is happening with them. I feel it in my body; I can see it in my eyes. This way I can assist them better. It is such a wonderful gift. However, it is a double-edged sword too.

Being an empath is like dealing with Arsenic. We know that Arsenic is a bad poison, but with homeopathic Arsenicum (Arsen I call it), we can heal mental restlessness, anxiety, burning pains, great thirst, perfectionist tendencies. You can also develop a tolerance when it is given on a continuous basis in small doses. Horses that are given small doses can have sleek and glossy coats. It aids turkeys with breeding and prevention of disease. Being an empath or a highly sensitive person is similar. While it is wonderful for healing, it can be terminal dealing with a narcissist without healthy boundaries. He dosed me continuously with his Arsen. Slowly I could take more and more.

The Oxford Dictionary's definition of Empathy (Noun): 'The ability to understand and share the feelings of another' (as in both authors have the skill to make you feel empathy with their heroines), whereas sympathy means 'feelings of pity and sorrow for someone else's misfortune' (as in 'they had great sympathy for the flood victims.')

Origin: Early 20th century: from Greek empatheia (from em- 'in' + pathos 'feeling') translating German Einfühlung.

I can absorb other people's emotions or physical ailments due to my sensitivities. I'm a good listener and I give all of myself to help others. This is very dangerous if we give our trust to those who are not deserving of it. A lot of times I was told I was just too emotional, to "suck it up", and toughen up. I cannot stand other people's suffering or hurting. It is in my DNA to help them in any way I can. I love to make people whole again. Now it is time to learn how my own thoughts and feelings are important and really matter. I need to be whole again to be able to flourish.

At the end of our five-year marriage and the seventeen years of our relationship, I had realized that my needs were not met. I was in constant fear of him. He threatened to leave me, to divorce me so many times. The last time it was on Valentine's Day, when his threats made my blood pressure go up to 200/120.

There was such a strong co-dependency with this man. He was supposed to be my forever partner and my knight in shining armor. I was panicking. What did I do wrong? Maybe if I do things better maybe, maybe... The more I tried, the more mistakes he saw. Nothing was good enough. I was expected to prepare a fresh three-course meal after work everyday. Oh, he helped me clean up afterwards. He was not satisfied with my cleaning the counter. So after I did it he re-did it - the same area, just to show me that I didn't do it right. "So, from now on you can do the cleaning as you do so much better job than me," I said to him.

Apparently, I didn't sleep right either as I had wrinkled the pillows. I was not supposed to do that. I felt criticized and made to feel inadequate, worthless. Everything I was doing was wrong. It happened daily. My work was Hocus Pocus? I mean magic, but he wanted all my income. He bothered me so much that I gave it to him just to stop the torture, day and night. When we went for a coffee he conveniently forgot his wallet and I had to pay for him. But the best was when he took me to a family restaurant and we were just sitting there and we couldn't order anything because it was too expensive.

Aside from the financial abuse he threatened me, intimidated me, constantly put me down emotionally, went into my email account and cleared it or opened my mails, listened in to my phone conversations or commented and joined in out loud when they were talking with me and not with him. He was overpowering and controlling.

What is abuse? When someone is using manipulation and fear to control and intimidate you, when someone makes you do things because of power and fear.

But how can that be? I'm an educated person and I thought I could handle it. It was done by slowly poisoning my life (Power of Control Wheel.) He could be so sweet and understanding. Sexually, he desired me constantly. "He really loves me. We have such a wonderful relationship," I would say to myself. At that time I didn't realized that he only loved himself and money. He was entitled to everything and really, I was his object. I didn't matter. I was just there to satisfy all his needs. To take care of him, clean, cook, have sex with. He loved to fall asleep at the TV. I couldn't wait for him to sleep, so I could go to my computer and study or do things that I had enjoyed. As soon as I would leave, he would wake up and yell at me because I was supposed to watch him fall asleep beside CNN as his mother used to do. Then the tension built. He was calling me names, or he paid no attention to me to punish me. I hoped maybe if I stayed there, maybe if I did more... maybe it is my fault. Then the abuse started, with the threatening and scaring. I was fearful but so tied to this man I couldn't even imagine leaving him (The Cycle of Violence). He told me I would be nothing without him. I was stuck, powerless, controlled and vulnerable. When you fear, you are feeling that you are not enough. You become powerless, defensive. You stop trusting yourself and your gut feelings. You become small, inauthentic. You forget who you really are. You are stuck in pain and suffering by your low self-esteem and by your small self. It was always my fault.

Gaslighting: Lying and manipulation, making the other person viewed as wrong and crazy.

Even though I had seen he was on porn or dating sites on the computer, he would explain to me that I didn't really see it right. He was so convincing, I believed him.

As a child, I hated to eat. My parents forced me to eat. Later on, food became my medicine. I had developed an eating disorder. Food gave me comfort, relaxed me and I didn't have to feel all my pain. Food made me happy. Food made me not feel the stress so much. It is still a journey for me to conquer.

I don't try to dance better than everyone else, I only try to dance better than myself
~Mikhail Baryshnikov

However, there were people – my husband, clients, and friends, who were Energy Vampires. They sucked my energy out so much that after being with them I needed to be on my own to recharge or to take a walk outside. I love nature as it fills me with unconditional love and energy. Energy Vampires and Narcissists love empaths, as they see them as victims who can easily be taken advantage of. Empaths however, are resilient and powerful – but they need time to heal after being a victim of a narcissist. After a year I'm still licking my wounds.

I thought I could handle him. He was familiar to me. He came from the same culture, he understood me. His mother was born the same month as me, and I could always confide in him. He seemed to have understood me. My psychologist friend begged me to leave him. I was so much in love. He offered me the fool's gold - financial security. I really thought I could handle him, but how wrong I was. Thinking back, I really should apologize to my friend for not listening to her. I could have saved so many years of pain, hurt, weight and humiliation.

Later on I had found out, that by my creating a sense of comfort, it just gave him more tools to manipulate me. He knew all of my insecurities and he knew how I worked. He looked at me with such a detailed eye, he dissected me. It was not that he really cared, it was to know how to humiliate me, how to embarrass me later on. The very last straw was when he said, "Things have to change and there are going to be new laws. You cannot have your parents over for dinner from now on." I felt he was trying to totally isolate me, keep me for himself.

He was right. There were new rules. The relationship had to end. It was the final breaking point.

> ...There is nowhere that a man can find a more peaceful and trouble-free retreat than in his own mind.
> ~Marcus Aurelius (Given equality, this quote really refers to all people – women included!)

I have to go back to the source, to Spirit. I have to rebuild myself. It is my inherent right to be loved and respected. It is not normal to fear every day or to walk on eggshells in an effort not to upset him or be embarrassed by him. I want to be authentic in who I am, what I believe in and who I want to spend time with, who I respect. I want a fearless life that is supported with love, understanding and mutual respect.

I used to be joyful, happy and full of laughter. Where did it go? Does anyone have the right to take my essence away? No, they don't. In mythology death is described as transformation, renewal. Something has to die to be reborn again. It is like in nature. In winter the trees, the flowers are dead or sleeping - just to wait for the spring to renew them and bud again in beautiful colors.

"The comeback is always greater than the setback."

Meditation has always been my salvation. I also give thanks everyday for my countless blessings. Because of its neuroplasticity, the brain is able to change the neuro-transmitters and establish new pathways. Dr. Daniel Amen has pioneered and documented with thousands of brain images how the brain is able to heal after PTSD, stress, obesity and brain injuries. It helped change the hopelessness and emptiness in me, my detachment from my husband's sadistic behavior, my inability to settle the separation and divorce.

I have realized the only thing I can change is my outlook, my thinking. I have forgiven him and I have forgiven myself. He doesn't know any better. Perhaps his childhood scars left him damaged so much. I forgive him but I do not forget his behavior towards me. Undoubtedly, my childhood scars had enabled him and myself to allow us to dance the dance of the abuser and the victim. I must move on, stronger and better, and armed with better boundaries so no one can hurt me the same way – ever again. I will now recognize the warning signs.

I have to change my mindset. I have to get back to my soul's purpose, be authentic, make an inventory and forgive. I'm worth it and I need to tell a new story. I believe the destiny is in charge. I surrender to it. It is unfolding in perfect timing and synchronicity. My soul has its map and plan, and I trust the spirit loves me. I'm whole again, I'm ready to step into my power and begin anew, even though it is scary for my ego.

I want to use this experience of Arsen to improve my emotional immune system and gloss my coat. I'm ready to be aligned with my truth and serve the world, but I need to heal first. I feel a deep spiritual bond, I am ready to grow, evolve, and nourish but remain aware of the true nature of humility. To surrender my troubles to Spirit and I believe I will be taken care of. If I can just help one person not to be so much in pain and broken as I was, I'm happy to be of service.

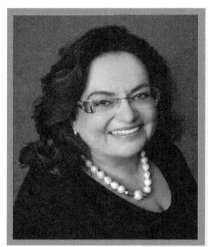

Andrea Judit Goldberger, RAC. DO (mp), DNM is a diverse Natural Health Practitioner and Therapist. An expert in Acupuncture, Natural Medicine, and Coaching in Natural Ways products. She is owner of The Gold Center for Parkinson and Natural Healing, Toronto, ON. Andrea is globally recognized in treating neurological conditions with Acupuncture, Osteopathy and Nutrition. Recipient of the Canadian Public Health Contribution Award (Aug. 2014) for Outstanding Services in Canadian Public Health, she is also the proud mother of Nicole and David.

Natasha Koss

From Rock Bottom I Found My Truth

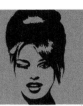

It's funny, life; the ups, downs, and around of it. 'Trust the Universe', a term I heard for the first time when I was in my early twenties. It stuck with me the rest of my life. I do believe in the power of energies, that similar souls travel together. That life happens to us and our attitude determines our outcome.

I live an ordinary life, I guess you can say. I'm married, work 40 hours a week and I take care of my family. I drive in rush hour traffic to and from work, prepare lunches, snacks and dinner. Weekends roll around, I scrub my toilets, take my kid to gymnastics and I think to myself, how did I get here? I walk through the many aisles of the grocery store admiring all the types of foods we are presented. I watch in awe at the families who grocery shop together as their children sit patiently in their shopping carts. They choose from the shelves filled with too much selection as a family unit like a coordinated dance. I could never bring my husband and daughter to the grocery store; he would compulsively buy whatever he saw, and my daughter would beg relentlessly for me to buy her candy. I would lose control and find myself overwhelmed buying nothing at all out of pure frustration. I would get home and be mad at them both. So, I choose to go alone. I got used to doing errands alone; it's a happy time for me. A time to reflect, breathe and think. I'm okay being with just me.

My life was not always this way. I used to be far more exciting. I worked in night clubs, went to the best parties and wore the latest fashions. I had dreams and aspirations in the art world and I knew a lot of interesting people. Then one day, none of the world I found myself in appeared fun to me anymore. The smoke and mirrors started showing its true colors. The fog lifted and the truth that I saw was not as glittery and sparkly as I once believed it to be. I started to crave the need to settle down and do something else, something different. It was a decision I have never regretted.

My so-called ordinary life is extraordinary to me.

Growing up I was always dramatic, outspoken, the lively one. Not much has changed over the years, except that life happened and has dimmed some of my early years' light. A broken heart, a lost job opportunity, a lost friendship, family troubles, issues with my daughter no parent should ever have to go through; the things that can happen in life, just happened.

Somehow out of the dark I always knew to search for the light. To find the reason in it all and push forward no matter what. Imagine for a moment that your life goes silent. You can't hear or see anything. What are the last things you would want to hear and see? I would want to watch my daughter dance and sing. She has the sweetest way of just floating as she dances and she sings like an off-key angel. I have come to treasure every moment with my daughter as there was a time when work left me with not much patience for her at the end of a busy day.

That steady light, though, almost went out. I almost and nearly touched the silence. I have been through some hard-times, and faced many an obstacle. But the ultimate of all fears came true in the summer of 2015. My daughter complained of a tummy ache. Nothing abnormal for a 4-year-old, but for us it was far from normal.

My daughter had asked me to bring her to the walk-in clinic. No ordinary 4-year-old, my child is intuitive and extremely intelligent, a star child I've been told on several occasions. It would make sense that she would find her own illness, she is that in touch with herself and her environment. The doctor from the walk-in clinic had felt what she thought was a swollen liver and recommended we get an ultrasound. After the ultrasound, I was sat down at a desk in an office in the hospital waiting room area, tissue box beside me with a specialist in tow. This did not feel right.

I was told that my daughter had a growth on her right kidney and that they were very concerned. Never in a million years did I clue in to what that even meant. We were then rushed to The Hospital for Sick Children. My daughter had to endure countless hours of more tests. It was so difficult to watch her cry and be afraid as they drew blood and put her in various machines. Large scary machines compared to my daughters fragile small frame. The truth was I did not fully understand what was going on, and I, too, was afraid. Confused and terrified, this was the hardest twenty-four hours of my life. The unknown is a very scary place to be.

How do you tell a family, a child, that they have cancer? The news touched my very being. It tested me as a mother, a wife, and as a woman. How could this happen to my healthy child? Cancer does not happen to kids, and not my kid! I was in complete shock. "We eat organic food, this is totally impossible," I told the doctor. "This is not happening, it can't be real." Her diagnosis made me question everything, especially my mothering skills. I felt like I had failed her, the guilt laid heavy on my heart and mind. But my biggest question: 'Why her and not me?'

The fact is, when it comes to childhood cancer, nothing we could have done would have changed this outcome. My beautiful, perfect, otherwise healthy, child had been diagnosed with stage 3 anaplastic Wilm's tumor - a kidney cancer that affects children up to the age of six. Wilm's has two types of histology's: the favorable (responds well to treatment); and, the unfavorable (does not respond well to treatment). In our spiraling world, rocked with nothing but bad news, the surgery was done to remove the tumor and the kidney, and pathology revealed that hers was of the worst and rarest kinds. She had the unfavorable histology. The bad news kept pouring in, the rivers and oceans of tears that I cried could have filled up Lake Ontario twice, the screams drowned the sound of a roaring engine.

I remember running down the halls of the hospital when they first told me the bad news needing to yell, scream and process, but could not find my air. I sobbed on the hospital floor, needing two nurses to get me back up and re-center myself. That was not the hardest part. The hardest part was walking back into my daughter's hospital room and acting like everything was okay. It took all of me not to shrivel up and die from the pain this diagnosis had on my heart and soul. But I am a mother, a strong woman, and I knew that everything that I had gone through up until this moment had prepared me for this. My daughter needed me at my best and I was ready to step up to the plate. I trusted the Universe now like never before. I found myself on my knees several times a day talking to God, begging and pleading for the cure. I found myself hanging on to every good luck charm, and listening to advice from every person who had information on pediatric cancer. I asked ten thousand questions and researched all I could on Wilm's tumor. I then became the expert. I became a real-life Dr. Mom. I knew the ins and outs of the chemotherapy, the names of all the medicines, the effects, and all the doses. I often impressed our oncologist with all I had been able to teach myself. Me, just a mom desperate to save my daughter's life.

I refused to let the light go out. I refused to even imagine for a minute that I would not see my daughter dance again or hear her sing in that oh so beautiful off key tone. I had the fight in me, and so did my daughter. I went from googling what CBC meant to ordering them myself, when I felt my daughter's counts were low and something might be wrong.

For reference, I'm the most anti-social, social person you'll ever meet. I am bubbly and outgoing, but have never been very good at making friends. I am a total home-body. I have been let down by a lot of people in my life. So in my adult years I chose to be kind and polite, but to always keep most people at arm's length. For fear of getting hurt, I have always lived in a glass house. You can see through, but the walls are always up. One of the hardest challenges I had to face early on in my daughter's diagnosis was to trust people. Teams of doctors and nurses, foundations and a lot of strangers were coming at us from every direction, and I had to trust them. My daughter's life depended on it. My survival in this journey depended on it. I now needed these people, I had no choice but to let down the wall and invite them in.

Trust the timing of your life is yet another important life lesson for me. It goes hand-in-hand with trusting the Universe. Three months before my daughter got diagnosed with cancer my father passed away. He was a sick man, but his passing was unexpected. We had a strained relationship; he was my hero growing up but then became a distant father. We grew apart. I could not understand him, and he could not understand me. The funny thing is, we had so much in common that we should have been best friends. My ego never let me get to that perfect place with my father, and, truth be told, neither did his. But I loved him so very much, even though I never told him. Never was that felt more on the day I found out that he died. Seeing his body lying in the hospital, just a shell, as his soul had moved on, I knew my father was gone and we had unfinished business. But also knew we would repair it now once and for all. I believe he is with me every day and especially during my daughter's illness. I trust that he passed away when he did to become my daughter's guardian angel. The time was right for him to go so that my daughter could stay.

The day my father died was also my birthday. I had not felt like doing anything that day. I had taken my daughter to her friend's birthday party and only wanted to come straight home. I turned down my husband's several restaurant dinner proposals. I just somehow didn't feel like celebrating me. When we got home I heard music playing in my house. I followed the sound and it led me to a doll. My daughters doll was singing a song with the verse, 'when will my life begin'. I could not make sense of it. This doll had never played on its own before and never played on its own again since. I was baffled but I blew it off and went to take a shower. I came downstairs and my husband gave me a look I had never seen before. He said, 'I must tell you something,' and that is when he broke the news. "Your father has passed away and you must get to the hospital right away." In total disbelief, I fell to my knees. My usually outspoken self could not even utter a single word. He was the man of nine lives. He had overcome so much in his life with his health issues and was doing well, but this time his heart just gave out.

Later that night, I had asked the doctor at what time did he pass, and it coincided with the time I got home and heard the song in my house. My father had come to me with a message, I could not shake the feeling he came to say goodbye through the doll. The song played over and over again in my head, "When will my life begin?" I just knew that was a message that I had to take in. What did it mean "my life beginning"? I am a mother, a wife, a career woman. How much more begun can I be?

Fast forward three months, I'm at Sick Kids (The Hospital for Sick Children) with my daughter fighting for her life. And at that moment, my life really began. The real me came out, the me I never knew was there. The me that had been building itself unknowingly for years. Hardship and pain from all the years passed, had turned into my ability to be the strongest mom I could be for my daughter, who needed me now more than ever. I felt my father's guidance every step of the way. We could not get on in the living life but we seem to be getting on great since his passing.

My daughter's treatment plan was aggressive. She endured 3 surgeries, 13 rounds of radiation, 12 cycles of chemotherapy, and had needed countless blood transfusions. We had many ups and downs, but she had the ability to overcome the odds. She had the ability to defy what was supposed to be, and remained playful and happy, even when her blood counts proved to be dangerously low. The doctors would often question how she could be so strong after having so much chemo. It all felt like something of a miracle, and perhaps it was.

As a mother, watching your child go through cancer and its treatments is nothing I would wish on anyone. But through it all I found my true strength; I found out that people - the right ones - can over exceed your expectations. Beautiful souls came to us. They offered us love and support; strangers whom we had just met wanted nothing more than to help us. I saw beauty on another level, humanity at its best. I owe a team of what were once strangers my endless gratitude for a life saved. The life of my one and only baby girl. I have learned the valuable gift of trusting people – that they are not all out to hurt me.

I spent countless hours on my knees praying, crying, wishing, and hoping for a cure, For a life better than this for my child. I laid beside her as chemo dripped into her tiny veins. At first it was scary. I trembled at the idea of chemotherapy and radiation, and, in fact, I still do. It's a hard price to pay. I often wanted to stop, and take her to be cured anywhere but the hospital. I researched so many types of cures. But the plan she was on came with extensive research, she had the best team of doctors on her side, and the cure was a real possibility. So when faced with life or death you only have one choice, we chose life.

Many times during treatment dealing with hospital stays, trips to the emergency, and in home isolation, I just needed it to end. I often wished I could be like everyone else, spending Saturday morning scrubbing my toilets and heading to the grocery store. These are things I do not take for granted anymore. These are things that if we are lucky enough to do, we must find gratitude in them. It's the little things, the tiny little things that truly matter. I now know that every let down in my life didn't make me weak and unworthy, but made me strong and deserving. It's in knowing the Universe has my back, and if I just pay attention to the signs I can lead myself to be the best me I can be. It's in knowing that everything has its time, and that time is the greatest healer and teacher.

It was not until I had been forced to face my biggest fears, that I had to face myself for the very first time. I could have easily chosen to bury my head in the sand and go through the journey depressed and afraid, present yet absent. Instead I stood up to the cancer, I opened all the lights and made sure only brightness, positivity, laughter, and love surrounded us. I made this time in our lives a happy and memorable one. I wanted my child to know that she was safe, loved, and that everything was going to be okay. Our mindset had a lot of power over us. Keeping the mind strong played a huge role in our journey. I never once made myself or my daughter the victims of our circumstances. Instead we had to find the reason in the ugliest places to prove we would get beyond this nightmare. Today my daughter is in remission. She is thriving, happy, and healthy. For me, my life has really truly begun. And it has nothing to do family or my career, but everything to do with clarity and my own sense of self. I can close my eyes and see my daughter dance and hear her sing, but I choose to open them and be present to her waving her arms around belting out her favorite song. I now know for sure that right here, right now, is where I am supposed to be. I live in the light of this journey, this amazing gift of life.

Natasha Koss has a background in fashion yet has always felt a strong pull towards writing. As a child before she could even spell, she was penning short stories and poems. The power of words have always fascinated Natasha as writing is her great escape. Author of the blog Selena's Journey and countless articles on the topic of living in positivity. A philanthropist, mother and wife, her passion for life lives within her words.

Gwenda Lambert

Now, I sing again

If you meet me, you would know right away I really don't have a problem speaking my mind. Yet the belief that I was supposed to take care of others, and that life was fleeting, in a literal sense, held me back for many years. I believed that no one was there to help me so I stopped asking for help – from anyone. That was the one that blew my mind. All it would take for the big bull to throw me clean into the wall was a simple statement, "Of course you should be supported."

One of the reasons my mind lived out this charade for so long is my, 'focus on the positive,' 'turn a positive into a negative,' reframing, as they call it in NLP (Neuro Linguistic Programming.) I knew there were millions of people who had it worse than I did. I grew up in a nice neighborhood. I had a roof over my head, food on my plate, was able to travel all over North America, visiting 35 states, 8 provinces and parts of Mexico all by the time I was 12. I had parents who loved history, and knowledge in general, which was, indeed, the best gift of all. But here is the part that matters. No matter what beliefs were going through my mind, by the end of this experience in extreme self-love, my soft place to land would be in my heart, and my gratitude for this adventure is something I say out loud every day. Most importantly, the very lie that my experiences were not so bad compared to millions of other people who had it worse off than me, did not take away from the fact that I needed to embrace and release the pain I had experienced. Until we can embrace all parts of us, we will never truly know love.

I am neither victim, nor survivor these are the threads that make the fabric of my life.
~Gwenda Lambert

Life is an ongoing series of experiences. Some are wonderful; like learning to scuba dive, and swim with the fishes; a night dive in Grand Cayman with a full moon as a super flashlight; a true belly laugh with friends; being completely connected in a moment of love that makes it impossible to doubt the existence of God; watching my nieces being born and grow; watching people I love grow and achieve their dreams; putting a smile on the face of a child. That I am able to put a smile on anyone's face, really, is a treat for me. The feeling that your heart was so big it was going to explode – awesome!!

Other experiences, like death, rejection, betrayal, violence, are not so wonderful. These times offered me an opportunity to continue keeping my heart open, forgiving those who hurt me. It was learning how to forgive those who truly wanted to break me. These times are heart-wrenching, and can overwhelm with shades of darkness. The breaking of a heart is painful, yet necessary to help us choose who we want to be, and how we want to treat ourselves, and others.

It was June 2013 when I was first diagnosed with Post Traumatic Stress Disorder. Later it would be called Anxiety Disorder with Aspects of PTSD as it was multiple traumas, others called it Complex PTSD. But what's in a label? I never much liked them. To me, it meant a whole bunch of unprocessed experiences stored in my mind and body that needed to be unpacked. While this was not my first rodeo, it was for sure the biggest bull I ever had to face. All the others seemed small in comparison. Yet they all allowed me to build my emotional muscle, training for the big event. You know, it doesn't really matter what the experiences are. For some, it can be a disease, like cancer, or the death of someone you love. For others, it may be a dysfunctional relationship, yet they all offer the same opportunities to learn about ourselves. I do not use words like victim, or survivor because I am still alive, still able to love all those around me, still able to do my best to make memories. I'm engaged whether I share a bus shelter with you for 15 minutes, or you are in my inner circle.

To thine own self be true.
~William Shakespeare

So what was the common thread between all those times where I chose life and love instead of fear and hate? Or worse; apathy and indifference?

First off, I needed a soft place to land. I needed to take myself out of harm's way, and take that first step to valuing myself enough to find out what makes me feel good, without artificial means. Early on that meant running, figuratively and literally; moving as far away from my childhood home as possible. I traveled as far as Bermuda, The Bahamas, Curacao, with a stopover in Barbados and Trinidad. It still wasn't distance enough from the baggage I carried with me. There were many suitcases to unpack. At one point in time, I had to take each one down and see what was inside. During this time of unpacking I continued to keep my connection to real tangible pleasures: physical activity; working out; riding my motorcycle, or bicycle; dancing; or, going to the beach. Water is special to me. One time I even drove to Cape Cod just because it had been too long since I had seen the ocean. It was a 12-hour drive. I love road trips.

Actually, before the last bull ride, all of my soft places to land had been stripped away, one by one. A mysterious shoulder/elbow issue took away my ability to even brush my teeth without pain. This meant no motorcycle, and no paddling for the competitive dragon boat team I was a part of. My sense of connectedness to my spirit was desperately missing. I felt like a balloon untethered and whipping around on the wind. My body was changing due to the lack of physical activity. I was longing for that soft place, yet know now that only by stripping it all away would I finally get to throw out the garbage that was locked inside.

What about you? Can you make a list of what makes you feel loved? Or grounded? Where is your soft place to land? More importantly, is it dependant on anything or anybody else? Or can you connect to it from wherever you are right now, even reading this passage?

The next step was commitment. I have had many times where I have had to choose life, choose love, and choose to try to understand others. My past saw me trying to figure out how I could work around them so they wouldn't hurt me. Many times there was no way out. It meant my beautiful mind took the worst of it and hid it away in this secret, locked room, and I would not recall it until the last bull ride.

Sometimes, it meant just praying for the end, not of my life, just praying for things to stop. None of this compared with the experience of the door of that room busting open, and the emotional unpacking of three specific events that would test everything I had ever known or experienced. Before that unpacking could occur, I had the no BS clause that had to happen between me and Me. I had to commit to myself at the deepest level I have ever experienced. That I was going to take care of business, and heal in no uncertain terms. I had a few terse conversations with the Universe, God, and any other entity that would listen. The most important of course was Me. There was a part of Me that was still on the outside, not believing it was safe enough to have dreams, or have her voice heard.

Does any of this ring true with you? Are you currently wooing the most important person in your world? When you look in the mirror, can you say I love you and mean it? Do you feel it?

See me, Feel me, Touch me, Heal me
~Tommy by The Who

You know the biggest problem with having conversations in your head is they have nowhere to go to be dealt with. They cannot take wings and fly to become something bigger. They cannot be seen in the light of day so you can decide if they will be a part of your story. If you cannot feel safe enough and courageous enough to say your thoughts out loud, how can you feel you are worthy to be heard?

The part I didn't expect in this wonderful experience is the amount of brain injury that it caused. Not being able to read, or to simply function in a manner that I had become accustomed, was scary. I had gone from never needing to write things down to not being able to hold a thought for 5 seconds. Every time I was triggered, it would take a month to get back on track. I had to focus on the moment.

Bearing witness is one of the most powerful and empowering things we can do for each other. There were three conversations on my journey that allowed me to get my story straight.

The first was with a dear friend at the end of May 2013. I had not yet had the formal PTSD diagnosis, and was convinced I had truly lost my mind. She would not let me isolate myself when I tried to back out of a long weekend trip we had planned. She listened for 3 hours to me crying tears from the very bottom of my soul, trying to make sense of how this happened in the first place. She held space when I was saying the words out loud for the first time. She also confirmed conversations I thought I had, like someone getting under my skin when it wouldn't normally bother me. This would become a lamp post I would hold onto when the storm was raging. This showed me the importance of a 'Write the SHITE out' journal. Sometimes, you just need to get the clutter out of your head in a 99-cent notebook, meant to be burned at the end of your journey.

Conversation two was after I had my diagnosis. This is specific to those who have experienced inappropriate sexual attention. This can be rape, or touching, grabbing, or even talking to you in a way that makes you feel unsafe. There doesn't need to be penetration to mess with your sense of safety and self. If you have had an experience like that and think it didn't leave a mark, I would truly ask that you let an experienced professional or moderated group help you make that call. In my experience,

116

there can be a difference in Childhood Sexual Abuse (CSA) involving someone who is outside your extended family, like a boy you have a crush on or a date, and someone you have to see at weddings, funerals, and other events on a regular basis. Standing up in these situations can cause rifts in families. It can also take you by surprise when you experience anger towards your parents as you may feel they didn't protect you. You may also find this transfer to other areas of your life if it is not addressed. When it is someone you may never have to see again, there can be that sense of space. Either way, the road to recovery can be a tough and emotional journey worth taking.

I was at a women's circle, a wonderfully safe space. It came to my turn to speak, and I happened to look at someone there who had experienced CSA. When I spoke to the loss of innocence that I experienced, she held my eyes, and said, simply, "Yes, I know." Though many had listened before, she knew what I meant. On a visceral level, it freed me in ways I cannot describe. It was so important to know that many of us experience similar things, and I was not alone. You are not alone.

The third conversation was when I had been triggered by a story in the news. Triggers lead to anxiety, crying, sleepless nights, and resulting reduced brain functioning. My goal was to roll with the triggers, climb deep inside and disengage them so that one day they would not sideline me anymore. A dear friend asked me questions and listened patiently when I reacted. She told me she had never been raped, and wanted to understand, without judgment. I knew she meant it. With my intention to heal, this again was a gift to express what was in my heart and head, and to work through the effects that by this point I feared would last forever. We cannot change people's minds with screaming. Until we own the 'react instead of respond' part, we will continue to yell. That rage, sadness, disgust, shame or loss of control, means you still have stuff to work out. You will never get to heal unless you confront the cause of the emotional expression. More importantly, we will never be able to move forward. Yes, there can be many of these conversations. Remember to keep your BS clause in check. Remember, too, when others are reacting, it is also worth taking a breath, and trying to see what else is behind their outburst.

It Takes a Village

This journey was mine, yet many helped in my process. I was blessed with great friends. I do want to add a caveat. Please don't be disappointed if during your healing, not all those around you can handle what you are dealing with. I find this especially with death and dying. It can trigger in them their own inability to handle such emotions. Please, love them anyway, knowing we are all on our own journey. Hold onto your friendship by staying away until you are on better ground. More importantly, remember, there are many people who will help if you ask for it, just as you would for them. I created a healing team.

I started with a therapist. I could write a whole book on all the different types of therapists, but I can tell you MSW's (Masters of Social Work) cannot officially diagnose. While I was correctly being treated for PTSD, in the middle of my crisis, I needed to go find someone else to officially diagnose me for insurance purposes. That was challenging, to say the least.

Please understand that your doctor is a member of your team and will focus on dealing with symptoms. It is important to understand that as a GP, they may not have experience to be able to help you with specific situations, and some specialists are exactly for a specific part, yet may not be able to help in other areas. That is why you need to remember you are a whole person; body, mind, and soul.

My naturopath was a doctor in Serbia before she came to Canada. She had this lovely biometric machine. My body is sensitive to drugs, so using this machine we were able to heal the adrenal/ hormone imbalance in my body, caused by stress, within 6 months using only drops.

My massage therapist was with me every step of the way. I would have a session with my therapist, and book a massage the next day to work it out of my body. My mystery shoulder issue was physically shaken out of my body years later. It seems it had something to do with the first assault. I'm telling you, in spite of the hard realities, this whole healing process was really fascinating. Thank God I am such a geek.

Equine Therapy is another wonderfully helpful modality, especially for PTSD as you connect with emotions that you may not be able to verbalize.

I hunted for Restorative Yoga with a smaller class size. Restorative Yoga deals with the parasympathetic nervous system allowing your body to relax whether it wanted to or not. Meditation is vital as well.

Network Spinal Analysis (NSA) utilizes light touches along the spine, coaching the nervous system to release stored tension and build strategies for responding to external stressors.

Energy work, such as Reiki, can help you break through blocks in your energy centers or Chakras. There are 7 main ones presented bottom to top: Root, Sacral, Solar Plexus, Heart, Throat, Third Eye, and Crown. The bottom three starting at the Root are grounding. The Heart is the center. The top three are connecting to Spirit.

I also saw an osteopath who works on the fascia and connective tissues which can hold the effects of trauma. I recommend this for anyone who may have experienced physical trauma, although they can help release emotional blocks as well.

One of the most fascinating experiences in this process was when I noticed a particular feeling that I wasn't grounded. I experienced a memory of having my head bounced off a wall, yet it had me across the room, clearly disassociated from the event. My RMT and Yogi helped me ground so by the time I was with my osteopath a few days later, her magic touch on my jaw and cheek landed me IN the memory. I was able to keep grounded while my body released what it needed to. This experience included the release of those tears from the depths of my soul. "Did you want me to stop?" she asked. No way. "Better out than in", as Shrek would say.

It has been five years on this healing journey. Add at least two years before that when I was already feeling the effects yet ignoring them. Now, I am finally at a place where I am confident enough to get out there. My triggers, or bounces as I like to call them, have gone from months at its worst, to just days of bearable anxiety. I have had the opportunity to embrace my lack of trust in men, something else I was unaware of, and gain confidence in being fully out in the world again.

I want to help people understand there are resources, places to go, and a soft place to land. I will continue to educate people of the different healing modalities they can use. I provide tools and insights on ways to understand yourself better so you can manage the way you react until you can learn to respond. After that, the world is yours to conquer. At my crisis point, I would hear, "they couldn't put Humpty together again" over and over again in my head. I was terrified that I would never be whole again - sane again. Well, here I am. I have tamed the bull. Humpty is together, albeit with gold-flecked super glue. But as they say in the world of Carnival, there is never too much glitter. If I can do it, you can too!!! No matter what the issue.

Now, I sing again. Much love now and always.

Gwenda Lambert,
Curator & Founder of Life Starts Now!
www.lifestartsnow.com

By deepening the relationship with yourself and ultimately, learning to love who you are; the sky is truly the limit! Gwenda helps individuals seeking to build self-resiliency, to accept themselves and their experiences. Gwenda brings a unique blend of healing and coaching modalities to her practice including: ntuitive observance, compassionate self-reflection, Socratic dialogue, and courageous curiosity. She is a certified NLP Coach and Practitioner, and has over 30 years of experience organizing, training and supporting people.

Michelle Main

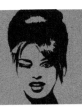

My parents separated when I was three months old. There were so many times in my life where I felt like an accident. I had no idea why I felt this way. It was nothing anyone had said or done, it was just in my head. In my opinion, happily married people don't have a baby and separate three months later if it was a planned pregnancy.

I was born asthmatic. In the book, You Can Heal Your Life, Louise L. Hay states that in babies and children, asthma is a fear of life – not wanting to be here. It goes on to say asthmatics, as the child ages, 'smother love. They have the inability to breathe for one's self. They feel stifled. They suppress crying'. My asthma appeared to be activity or allergy induced, but I wonder if it wasn't related to my sense of not belonging. Sometimes it was worse than others. I managed mostly with allergy medication and different puffers that weren't very effective. When I was twelve, they booked me to go to The Chest Clinic at The Hospital for Sick Children. They prescribed asthma medication that made me so sick. It was really hard on my stomach and took a lot of getting used to.

I lived with my mom and stepdad during the week and I went to visit my dad on weekends. He usually called Thursday nights to confirm arrangements to pick me up after school each Friday. One Thursday he didn't call, so my mom suggested that I call him. When I reached him, he told me that he wasn't feeling well. I suggested that I wasn't feeling well either, so maybe we could not feel well together. As always, 'Daddy's little girl' got what 'Daddy's little girl' wanted. Daddy came to pick me up. He had to work on the Saturday and I told him I would go with him. My dad had suffered a heart attack at age 38 and was then 43 years of age. I remember us at his work, sitting on a pallet in the warehouse leaning on each other. We both truly felt like sacks of shit. I swear, we were holding each other up. That night, coming in from the car, I ended up throwing up before reaching his apartment. He held my hair while popping a Nitro under his tongue. He had been having bad chest pains all week. He drove me home on the Sunday night and, as always, we held hands. Little did I know that would be my last touch, my last ride, my last weekend, my last everything, with this man who was my world.

That week, after my visit with my father I was back at the Chest Clinic for follow up. It was a fun day. We met up with my mom's best friend, Pearl, and my Uncle Doug was with us, too. We were playing games on the way back from the hospital, making phrases out of the letters on license plates of cars around us. My stepdad's mother had been babysitting my siblings. She didn't speak English very well, and when we arrived home she blurted out to my mom, "I think her dad is dead!"

I often didn't understand her, but I certainly understood that! I yelled, "No!" I remember Three's Company was on TV in the living room.

That was my favorite show. It was a bit of a diversion while I waited for confirmation that my dad was okay. It was the episode where Larry was in the coffin. My mom called the phone number that was left and got the dreadful news that yes - my hero, my buddy, my Daddy - was dead. My mom looked at my Uncle Doug and nodded her head 'yes'. I screamed "NOOOO!" "NOOOOOO!" And burst into tears.

I went to run, but my Uncle Doug reached out and grabbed me and squeezed me so tight, and just held me. I collapsed in his arms and truly felt like I was going to die. I had so much pain in my heart. I truly believed that I could actually feel my heart break. That really was the worst day of my short life. My face broke out in hives instantly. The following days were almost unbearable. I couldn't imagine life without him. Seeing him lie there, lifeless, covered in make-up, he didn't even look like himself. And he was so cold. I kept rubbing his makeup off because I kept hugging and caressing his face asking him to please come back to me. I just wanted to go with him.

There wasn't a dry eye in the funeral home. Everyone felt saddened and helpless; they had no idea what to do with me, or for me. I still miss him so much. I have been to therapy and experienced many other modalities to help process this tragic event. In writing this, I realize that it's definitely something that still needs work.

My spine started collapsing that year. I had a very noticeable curvature and a lot of pain. I was so self-conscious of clothing, especially bathing suits, that showed the unnatural look of my back. I felt so ugly and so out of place. Other girl's looked so perfect, and I was deformed. And, naturally, children were cruel and teased me about it. There was a guy

I liked. He made fun of me by putting a life jacket under his shirt and hunched over and said "Yes Master" and limped while hunched over. I was humiliated, and crushed. Life is interesting. He later developed Scoliosis.

Many family doctor and specialist appointments offered conflicting opinions. The last specialist we saw proposed surgery. My stepdad wanted yet another opinion, but he was told there was no one else to go to; we were at the top tier of specialists. We went with his opinion to operate on an 84-degree curvature of my spine. The surgery outcome could be full recovery, paralysis, or death. I had to beg my mom to let me have the surgery. I now have steel rods in my back, officially called Harrington Rods. The condition is called Kyphosis, similar to Scoliosis. Scoliosis, however, is an "S" curvature, whereas my curvature almost folded me in half. When I walked into a room, I came in head first, hunched over.

It was awful. I felt so ugly and self-conscious. My pre-op curvature measurement was 82 degrees. I had collapsed 2 more degrees in 24 short hours. I was wheelchair-bound, and unable to have children in my future at this rate. As they were wheeling me to the operating room, I was waving at my mom telling her that I loved her. I said, "Remember, if anything bad happens, I wanted this surgery." If I ended up paralyzed or dead, I didn't want her to feel guilty. Although, now that I'm a parent, I know she would have anyway, regardless of what I said.

Years later, these two traumatic incidents were linked through a Reiki Master. On her questionnaire, it came up that my dad had died when I was very young. She concluded that because of losing my 'support system' (my dad), I had to have support physically installed by having my spine surgery. I was blown away! It made total sense to me. It was also a pivotal moment when I started to look to alternative healing instead of conventional medicine.

From about the age of twelve, after my dad died, I started worrying about my weight, too. I guess it was my age. I was looking to wear tighter jeans. I tried to eat right and exercise. In high school I bounced from diet to diet and I exercised compulsively. In my lifetime, I'm sure I have lost hundreds, if not thousands of pounds. The sad thing was that when I started this craziness, I weighed just 117 lbs and was 5 foot 3 inches tall. My friends were telling me that I was fine; I didn't need to lose weight. Why was I obsessing this way? Addictive behavior is why; people making fun of me, boys teasing me, trying to fill a void.

I do have a highly addictive personality that has showed up in several ways. I can overdo almost anything: food, exercise, meetings, work, spending money. There is no gray area for me. Everything is black or white; all or nothing.

At a young age, I had a very entrepreneurial spirit. My dad used to take me into work and show me the air conditioned office where the secretaries worked. He told me he did not want me to work like he did, with a hard physical job, and no air conditioning. My mom worked for the government and I remember how beautiful she looked going to work. That's what I wanted. I used to watch 'The Young and the Restless' on TV with my mom, and when my friends or cousins would come over to play, I would be at my stepdad's desk pretending to be Ashley. I wanted to own a family business like her. Today that fantasy is my reality. I own my own business; my son helps me out, and also has his own business.

One day, the ladies from Avon came knocking at our door and tried to recruit my mom, but she wanted nothing to do with it. I was not old enough, so I begged her to sign up so that I could do it. She did, and I loved it! I remember delivery days, sitting on the kitchen floor with all the products sprawled all over the floor and putting my customer's orders together with such pride.

Problems arose soon after I started my business when the lovely little old lady across the road became my customer. I always ended up alone with her husband while she went to get the money to pay me for her order. He always looked at me in a way that made me very uncomfortable. Somehow he always managed to get me into the back yard, and he would grab me and hold my arms and grind on me from behind. He would also put his hands up my top and down my pants. It felt so gross! I would struggle to get away and just couldn't. This happened far too many times. One time I went to deliver her order and she went in to get the money and, as always, I was all alone with him. While looking me up and down and almost drooling, he said, "Oh Sweetie... would I ever love to lick you between the legs." I almost puked. That, however, was what broke my silence. I went home and told my parents.

These people were clients of my stepfather, who was an accountant. He had done their taxes for years. He jumped out of his chair and was going to go across the street and confront, or kill him. My mom wouldn't let him go. I wish he had, because it turned out that I wasn't the only person he had done this to. Silence is not the answer. I remember hearing that he had molested a friend of my sister's right on the driveway in front of his house. There was a witness, but they did not get involved or stop him.

I wish I could say that was my only experience with molestation, but that's not the case. We used to go visit family where my own cousin would pull me in tight and go up my top. The lasting effects of these traumas are that I need to be approached from the front. I cannot be woken up in the night or I start swinging my fists and defending myself. Those memories and feelings affected me throughout my marriage. I gained weight, and I think it was to protect myself from such attention. Over the years, I have also been in multiple car accidents and sustained many injuries. I also have chronic fatigue syndrome and fibromyalgia. I have been in pain for twenty years, twenty four hours a day. Movement is limited and there have been side effects from medication.

At a business networking event that I was supposed to be hosting I couldn't even gain the strength to stand up and introduce myself. I knew at this point that something had to be done.

Due to the way I had been feeling, I dragged myself to the walk-in clinic. They decided to do a chest X-Ray due to difficulty breathing and chest pain. It showed a seven centimetre fat pad near my heart that was causing the pain. I freaked out and could only think, 'Oh my God! I am going to die young like my dad!'

From that business networking event, there was someone promoting a nutritional cleansing system. I committed to it and in my first nine days,

I released seventeen-and-a-half pounds and twenty-one inches. I was impressed and excited and felt better. My brother was getting married soon, and I decided that I was going to keep going and lose fifty pounds before his wedding.

Well, I didn't lose the fifty pounds, but I did lose forty-eight-and-a-half pounds, and forty-nine inches. Close enough! I was thrilled with my results. People complimented me on how great I looked. It was nice to be complimented and to achieve success. I looked and felt way better than I had for a long time. I had even implemented an exercise routine after the loss of my first twenty-five pounds, and I hadn't exercised in years.

The excitement was short-lived. I don't know if you have ever attended an Italian wedding, but let me tell you the food is phenomenal! You know what is even better than the wedding? The leftovers! We were sent home with the leftover food and the leftover cake. I decided to take a two-day break from my lifestyle change. I was in my glory! I would have some pasta, then some cake, then more food, and more cake. It was divine!!!

Unfortunately, that two-day break went much longer.

It was the summer of 2012 and my life was unmanageable. I would eat to the point where if I swallowed one more bite I would throw up. I hate to admit it, but that was my cue to stop eating. Back then, when life didn't go my way, I went out of my way to eat large quantities of the worst quality food. I would even beg and manipulate people to go on a junk food or fast food run for me. If they refused, I would be the biggest bitch until they caved in and got me what I wanted. Oh the insanity! And the cruelty. Looking back, I feel so horrible at the way I treated my husband when I was on a food bender.

And it wasn't just food that was addictive. All through school, teachers would write, 'Michelle lacks comprehension' on my report cards. I hated to read. I didn't get good grades. I didn't like school. I turns out that I was just bored and uninterested in what I was reading. As an adult I love to read! I also comprehend what I read. I choose what I want to read, and those are books that can help me and thoseI love. I love books! I love used books! I buy books about natural health, self-help, business, personal development, weight loss, aromatherapy, and more! I have morebooks than a small town library! One time, I was at Goodwill store and there were books from OA (Over-Eaters Anonymous). I thought to myself, 'What the hell? I'll grab the books and maybe someday I will read them.' I had attended a meeting when I was in my early twenties. I remember sitting there, listening to people 'sharing'. I thought to myself what the hell is wrong with these people? It is so depressing here. People were crying and complaining. When the meeting finished, I was told to 'keep coming back.' I thought, 'Not on your fucking life! If I come here week after week, I will jump off a bridge.' That was my perception. Not necessarily how it was. But I never went back.

That summer, for my son's birthday and we had bought a cake for 45 people. Three quarters of the cake was left. I ate it all and was standing at the door with my purse and car keys in hand, ready to go to the grocery store to buy another one. There was no logical reason why I would do this. What in the hell was wrong with me?! I was hell bent on this path of self-destruction. It was at this point that I realized I had a problem. I went looking for the OA books that I had bought from Goodwill. I read them that weekend and looked right away for a meeting.

I went to the next available meeting in the closest town. It was on a Tuesday. I felt so welcome and so at home. The timing was finally right for me. I had asked a friend of mine to come with me because I was so scared and embarrassed. There was a guest speaker that night. It's like she was telling my story. I looked at my friend, my eyes filled with tears, and I stood up to leave. He grabbed my hand tight and pulled me down and kept me in my seat. I'm glad he did. I listened to what people said and watched what they did and I agreed to come back the following week. They started going around the table and introducing themselves. It was my turn. I was scared to death to open my mouth, but somehow, I managed.

"Hi… My name is Michelle. I'm a Compulsive Over-Eater and Food Addict." Seriously? I'm one of those people? Yes! I definitely am one of those people, and I am so grateful that I found my way into the rooms of recovery. I had found people that were messed up like me. I wasn't glad that they were messed up. But I was glad that I found people who understood me, accepted me, who I accepted, and who could relate to me, and who I could relate to. I no longer felt alone.

My first abnormal food behavior came to me as I progressed through recovery. I had a vision of a gathering where steak was served for dinner.

I remember going around the table and asking everyone for the fat off their steak. I ate it all! No idea why I would want to, or why they let me. I remember people laughing. Was it for attention? Today, I find that repulsive and would never do it again. Gag!

On September 6th, 2017, I will be five years abstinent. To me that means five years with no cake. I didn't think I could go five minutes. A friend in the program helped get me through, minute by minute, then day by day. Then months. Then years. I have changed many bad habits and many other things along the way. I am very proud of myself for making 'me' a priority and for continuing. I honestly thought I would give up on myself and quit.

As I mentioned, I also love to shop. I was looking for that missing something from my life. I was desperate. I started on a personal development journey, buying self-help books, attending seminars, and taking courses. But I bought more than I could possibly attend, or read. Yes, another addiction! At least this one is a good one. A little over a year ago, I purchased an online course for NLP (Neuro Linguistic Programming.) This program, like so many others, sat on a shelf (this one on my 'email shelf'). I have all kinds of folders in my email for such things. I did open it. I got completely overwhelmed and closed it down. And there it sat for more than a year.

My husband and I are currently separated. Although it is mostly my fault, I am still broken. I was sinking, sleeping all the time, crying when I was awake. I couldn't cope. I needed help, and thought, 'Where the hell is that online course?!!!' I went looking through my email files and found it. I opened it up and, again, was overwhelmed, but I mustered up the courage to leave it open and start. I've seen a quote that goes something like this, 'You don't have to complete the entire staircase - you just have to take the first step.' I was very proud of myself for seeking help when I needed it. And I actually finished the course and am now a Certified NLP Practitioner! Remember I mentioned that I didn't do very well in school? I was amazed when I passed this course. I am so excited at how much I was able to help myself first, and how much I was able to overcome; and now being able to help others. There is always more - to learn, to experience, to share, but here are some points to remember:

- If our birth is planned or an accident, we are meant to be here, and can do great things.

- Never take your health for granted.

- Treasure your loved ones and spend as much time with them as possible.

- Get help to work through your stuff at the first sign of trouble.

- You are good enough. Love yourself exactly as you are, right now in this moment.

- Love what you do for a living so it doesn't feel like work.

- Set your goals and do what it takes to achieve them.
- Don't let what others say define you.

- Invest in yourself. You will get the greatest Return On Investment.

- Everything! I mean Everything in moderation.

- Celebrate your successes.

- Be kind to yourself and others.

- Live with passion.

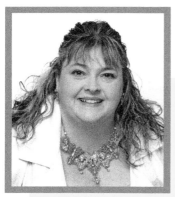

Michelle Main is the Founder of U Can Change Your Life. Specializing in a Healthy Lifestyle, Wellness and Cleanse Coaching. Her passion is helping others Change Their Life. Recently Certified in NLP (Neuro Linguistic Programming) she was able to overcome addiction, release fears and trauma. Michelle is an Entrepreneur, a Philanthropist, Networker, Master Connector and Motivational/Inspirational Speaker. Due to her love for nature, she is all about natural products, natural health and green products. Michelle is a mom to her beautiful and amazing son Carson.

Claudine Pereira

Life Lessons learned from the school of hard knocks!

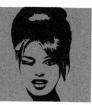

What would I tell my Younger Self?

Lesson 1 You don't use anything you learn in school in real life!

> "Dearly beloved, we are gathered here today to get through this thing called life."
> –Prince

I spent 16 years in the UK school system and quite frankly I did not enjoy school. School was about having a good laugh with your mates, or bunking off down to the chip shop. A typical primary school education at my Church of England school in the little town of Reading, England consisted of morning Eucharist and prayers and then assembly. We actually spent most of the time laughing at the Head Master and his squeaky shoes. We really loved him. (Insert happy memory here). Although we all used to run from him as no one wanted to end up in his office for a good dose of the cane. Oh yes! Corporal punishments were real. After our morning milk, which I seem to recall giving to my mate to drink (yuk), it was off to classes or swimming. Swimming! Sounds exciting right? But check this out. We had to walk across the school field in the cold damp foggy British morning air, grass full of dew, in just our bathing suits. And off into the cold pool we went! Smashing! My Mother couldn't understand why I was always sick.

Upon reflection, school didn't equip me to deal with life's tough rude awakenings; relationships, family, mental illness, racism, sickness, or even motherhood. Perhaps one of the major reasons I hated school was the racism. I had nowhere to turn. My family is from the West Indies and my gorgeous black Grandmother used to do the school run with my sister and I. "Why is your Nan black?" I would hear. I had mocha-colored skin which led the kids to say cruel things like "Bloody Paki - so ugly," or "Rubber Lips." Back in the 1980's having fat lips wasn't a popular look; thin lips were the fashion. I really couldn't understand what was going on, but it hurt. I have to say I get a bit of a giggle now when women are paying for dark skin and Botox to enhance their lips! Who's having the last laugh now?

Already a target for racism I made things even worse by killing the school hamster. I grew up in a cold moldy box room of my Grandparents' home. My room was so cold that when I took the school hamster home for Easter weekend he was stiff as a board the next morning. Easy fix - buy another dude, right?! It turns out new hammy hamster was vicious and bit the kids. Give me my cats any day!

The favoritism from the teachers was the best. The smart kids used to sit at the 'middle table' in class. My cousin, who was super smart, sat at that table. I couldn't understand why I wasn't there. I was 11 and thought I was smart, too. I seem to recall quitting school at that point. No one really knew why; not even me. I just felt unhappy all the time. After conversations and social worker chats, I went back to the same class but this time I was placed at the middle table by the old bird teacher who used to stir sweetener in her coffee with the end of her pen.

Secondary school wasn't much better. Half the time was spent hanging around the back of the bike sheds with the smokers, luckily a habit I didn't pick up. I did pick up some others, like skipping classes. I avoided gym class. How is running in the cold damp foggy English morning going to get me through life?

I had to take 2 buses to school. The 4:00 p.m. bus from town was one to avoid. From bullying to egg throwing it was a fearful experience! At the age of 14 when I met my first love, everything changed. Life was finally worth living! Getting picked up from school in your boyfriend's car was a thing! I can still remember the day he came to watch me dance in the middle of the school field in my all-in-one blue cat suit! (More about him later.) All I wanted to do was see him and take my dance classes.

I don't dwell on the past. Did it suck? Yes, but I'm so blessed to be able to use my bad school experiences to help others, whether it's my clients, or my daughter or her friends. Not everyone copes well with their past and that's where I love to help others. This is what is lacking in our kids today; good old fashioned grit and determination. When I ran into problems as an adult could I have referenced school? "Well self, why don't you just solve your relationship problem by applying what you learned in Grade 12 English class. Hmm, maybe not. OK, off you pop! Carry on." Or, "I'm so proud of you, self, that you can use the Pythagorean Theorem from Grade 11 Math to figure out the cost of buying versus leasing a car! Ha! Laughable!

When I went back to school as an adult, I then began learning with passion and purpose. Leading and guiding others through life has become my passion and gift. So thank you school for that cruel, ugly life lesson because it turned out to be a beautiful gift!

Lesson 2 Be Authentic and be YOU!

"Be yourself; everyone else is already taken." ~Oscar Wilde

This one is huge. I spent many years not knowing who I was. The real me. I was walking on egg shells and adapting my personality to suit others needs; from family, to friends, and my employer. I was a lost soul. I had several sides to me, acting and even thinking differently depending who I was around. A big people pleaser, I had a hard time saying no. And guess how I ended up? Bloody exhausted. A right disaster! Growing up in my grandparents' home I lived in a house full of adults that were fighting and arguing all the time, so I withdrew. I loved them dearly, but it wasn't a great environment for a child. The only time I was happy was when my cousins came to visit and we would play our ritual musical game of Miss Wonder Horse in the hallway. Other than that, I would play with my cat and sit in my cold room. Not good.

And so the treading on egg shells started in my life. Fear of confrontation, or asking for anything I needed trickled into my adult life; unable to say 'no' to anyone, running myself ragged, pleasing everyone, but not myself. At the age of

13 I wouldn't even ask for anything in a store, "Mummy can you ask for me?" It wasn't until I ended up in counseling many years later that I discovered the conflict in my childhood home was the underlying issue for my problems. I nearly fell off my chair. Who would imagine adults arguing, yelling, or ignoring one other would impact me so much?

My Mother didn't know what to do with me, so she took me to dance school. It was the best thing that ever happened to me. Dancing saved my bacon. "Oh Mrs. Pereira, Claudine's posture is dreadful, but let's see what we can do with her." I remember listening to that and thinking, 'what on earth is posture?' Duh! No wonder I wasn't at the middle table! So I started to blossom and speak up. Glimmers of me came out. Throughout my life, and even today, dancing has been my hope, my saving grace, a place where I can be someone else; stepping every time outside of my comfort zone. Most of my fellow dancers had major body image issues. But I didn't. Until one day in the middle of a ballet class, the teacher told us that, 'some of us in class are getting too wide in the hips.' There were only two of us in the class! My friend was skinny as a rake, so who does that leave then? Me. I was upset. It hurt, so I tried to starve myself skinny, avoiding my Grandmother's signature fried chicken. One of my Aunts actually asked my Mother if she was starving me. It amazes me how careless people can be with their words, to have no concept of the impact it has on the receiving person. Today, I have no clue what I weigh. I am proud of my West Indian curves, aka 'duck disease', as my Grandmother used to call it. So there! This is me.

The other place where I couldn't be me was at the office. Conforming to the demands of a corporate career changed me. I wasn't equipped to handle challenging conversations with the 'higher ups', so I had to pretend. 'Fake it till you make it' in the Shark meetings. You would either sink, be sunk, or get eaten alive, or swim! Perhaps it was my fear of confrontation? Don't get me wrong I really loved my job. I lived for my employees; they were my life there. It wasn't until I left that I reflected with my coach and realized I did a job for twenty years that wasn't me; it was not aligned with my values. Wow! Another falling off the chair moment. Huge! I had never even considered values when I was looking for a job. I thought I just needed a job. Now I will not do anything, or be around anyone that does not alig with my values. The beauty of that experience is that it has helped me enormously in my business today. If I hadn't lived that torture, I wouldn't be of service in my business and able to help others that have had similar experiences.

That was a turning point in my life. It took me a good year to figure out who I was. Me. The real me. Prayer, yoga and meditation saved me. I spent so much time conforming to other people's points of views and opinions over the years, "Yes, Sir." "No, Sir." "Three bags full, Sir!" Well no more, the worm has turned! As a business owner I am blessed to be authentic in my business. What you see is what you get. I no longer need to tailor myself to others' expectations. You don't like it, well that's too bad! So many others suffer from this, and I am now in the fortunate position to be able to help. So, be you! There is only room for one! You will feel much lighter for it.

Lesson 3 Pay attention to everyone you meet; they may change your life

> "They're the people that you meet, when you're walking down the street. They're the people that you meet each day."
> ~Bob - Sesame Street

I didn't understand for a very long time there is no such thing as a chance meeting. Boy was I missing out! But seriously have you noticed that sometimes people just pop up in your life and bring amazing gifts? I don't mean material ones. These gifts can take many forms; connecting you to business opportunities, other likeminded people, something new to learn. The opportunities are endless if we have our antennas up. Are we paying attention to those who cross our path?

Once I was working out in Western Canada and made friends with a wonderful homeless man who I nicknamed One-Eyed Jack. He literally had one eye, and he told me the gory story of how he lost it! It was an awesome conversation in a bus shelter, one that would have a lasting impact. I bid him farewell and continued to walk up the hill to find my dining spot for the night. But I couldn't get him out of my mind. So I spun around, and went back to find him. I invited him to dinner and we sat down to eat much to the stares and the shock of the fellow restaurateurs'. Dude needed a meal and I was in a position to help. Every time I returned there, I would look him up. Just to see his smile when I came to see him made my day One-Eyed Jack was sent to give my corporate self a wake-up call. We have so much to give back. He was a lesson in humanity. I recently read the book,

"The Alchemist" By Paulo Coelho. I encourage you to add it to your reading list. In reflection we are going through life at a rapid pace, always focused on the end result, the end goal. The one big thing. So when we finally get there, then what? How about taking time to see what really is happening to us day to day. Who are we meeting and why are they in our life? What is making us happy? Material things, money, power? Ask yourself if you are receiving messages. Are you paying attention to them and paying it forward? We need to stop and smell the roses.

Lesson 4 You will always remember your first love; the good or the bad!

"Dream Lover come rescue me."
–Mariah Carey

Who has never forgotten their first real love? I know I haven't. Even though as a teen I was naive, he made me feel like no one else mattered. He was a bodybuilder, and worked at my dance school. I was 14 years old, say no more! There was a 3 year age difference which, at that age, was huge. My heart was innocent and pure and he broke it. Sigh. He is responsible for my love of old music. At weekly visits to his parents we would listen to the old 50's and 60's classics.There were no cell phones, so we would write letters to each other as a means of keeping in touch. Old fashioned right? Did I mention before I used to get giddy when he would pick me up at school in his old Daf car? He always had a cute, little gift, or token for me. One memory is he engraved my name on a gorgeous identity bracelet which I wore for years after. Times were good.

Tragedy struck. His best friend from birth was killed in a stabbing outside a club in town. Sigh. I will never forget waking to the news on the radio. It was such a tragic time in our lives; the whole town went into mourning, as did we. After that he changed. I found out he was cheating with a woman right under my nose at the dancing school. In my rage, I tried to shove him in the canal in town. Yikes! Was that me? As much as this ended with my heart broken, there is a small part of me that hasn't forgotten how he awoke my heart, and I would perhaps still go giddy and weak at the knees if I saw him again... well, maybe not!

So many people I speak to are having major relationship issues. Many put up with bad behavior, violence; it is sad to watch. Be careful who you chose as your first love, or any love as a matter of fact. They become part of you. They stay with you. Good, bad, or indifferent, as we age we become more sentimental and these memories creep back into our lives like a bad smell. So choose wisely, think before you give your heart away as it may come back to bite you later on in another part of your body!

Lesson 5 You're known by the company you keep

> "Never wrestle with pigs. You both get dirty
> and the pigs like it."
> ~George Bernard Shaw

Inspirational guru Tony Robbins says,"Who you surround yourself with is who you will become." And it is so true. My younger self would never have believed this, but upon reflection, my friends were a huge influence on me and my people pleasing personality. I lived day-to-day, surrounded by drinkers and people flying by the seat of their pants literally. I chose the wild side of life, going down the pub, clubbing and never caring what tomorrow brought. During my early career in England, we would live for a Friday night, and go out and spend any little money we had. I came from a poor home, so money was super tight. I was hanging with some so-called friends that would mock me by whispering loudly to each other as to why I wasn't buying the next round. I just couldn't afford to.

If I had continued on that path I'm not sure what would have become of my life. Instead, I chose to upset the apple cart and change my life. When I moved to Canada I made two super solid friends that are in my life to this day. Still dealing with my people pleasing self, I was still attracting time-suckers, users, and so-called friends that would try to drag me down to their level with their problems and negativity; energy zappers. I remember one of my friendships others would comment on saying, "Wow, she is nothing like you!" Think about some of the friends you have had, or may still have. Do you ever notice how you slowly become like them? We are greatly influenced by those closest to us. Jim Rown says, "You're the average of the five people you spend the most time with. "Have you ever noticed the moment you find a new friend, or enter into a new relationship how this makes you feel? Especially if the person is full of life and positivity, it becomes contagious. Since I chose the path of being an entrepreneur, I now surround myself with people who are moving in the same direction as me, with similar values. It has become a huge game-changer. Once my antennas went up and I realized I was being used, I set my boundaries. In the past I would self disclose my deepest fears and secrets only to be bitten in the 'you-know-what'. Now self-disclosure is a choice and there has to be a purpose. I made peace with not having a ton of friends, just those few that would always be there for me, holding the space without judgment and always with love always. You know who you are!

Lesson 6   The older you get the less you will care about what people think about you (really)!

"A lion doesn't concern himself with the opinion of a sheep."
~George R.R. Martin

Growing up in a West Indian household was interesting. It was full of judgment and finger pointing. "Girl, you too skinny. "Girl, you put on weight?! "Why you cut your hair so?" I was always worrying and wondering what people thought of me. Are they going to like me? Is my hair right? My make up? I hid behind it, because I really didn't know who I was. I always thought people were talking about me, so I a ways had to over-impress. Again, enter the people pleaser. This trickled into my work, friendships, and relationships. Once I overheard female Managers at my workplace talking about what I was wearing and judging me. These employees were my leaders, so what could I do? Try harder to dress better, neater, nicer. That would make them like me right? Wrong! Just like school, there are also bullies in the workplace. Once I turned 40 something shifted. I started to worry less and less about what people thought about me. And now I couldn't give a rat's behind about what people think. Take me or leave me, I am who I am (I think that's a song)? Now there is also a fine line to this. I do care about what some of my loved ones think and my clients, however the comments and finger-pointing you experience growing up will bother you less and less as you age. My wonderful dance teacher has a saying, "Their problem is not your problem. What people think and feel about you or anything else isn't your problem so don't own it. " When you really think about it, that is powerful stuff.

Lesson 7   Work on yourself inside and out

> "If you don't make time for working out, you'd better make
> time for illness."
> ~Robin Sharma

I used to rely on other peoples' approval of me, I'm sure you get the picture by now. If they were happy I was happy, or so I thought. Friends, work, family, I was only happy when I made others happy. Crazy, right? I lost myself and had no clue who I was anymore. Saying no was like a poison word. I would say yes to everything and everyone. Seriously? Now that's exhausting. The only person that can really make you happy is, guess what? YOU! Yes, look in the mirror; you and you alone can bring happiness. The stress of it all made my hair start to drop out, body rashes, allergies to hair products. I had to do my inner work. When I left my corporate career, I started the task of working on me. Yoga, meditation, prayer, and acceptance of the person that I am! Not what others expected of me.

Part of that is to workout and sweat! I know, I know, coming from the person who used to skip gym class in England to go eat fish and chips in the precinct is talking about working out. I have been a CrossFit addict for 9 years. The 6:00 a.m. class is my life. My day isn't complete if I don't go. My guru

Robin Sharma preaches about the '5:00 a.m. Club' and how it is a game changer. He is so right. The days when I am up early to workout I feel like a champ, just like Rocky Balboa, ready to take on the world. Working out and eating well has made a huge impact in my life and continues to be. Is it easy? Of course not, but this is where discipline comes in. Maybe those early hard days in England paid off after all. Guaranteed it will change your life, if you allow it to.

Lesson 8   It's OK to follow your dreams!

"All our dreams can come true if we have the courage to pursue them."
~Walt Disney

How many of you fell into your career? Was it ever the job or career you dreamed about as a kid? Most likely not. Growing up I wanted to be a veterinarian until I realized what that would entail. (Moving quickly past that.) Next it was a flight attendant because I wanted to travel. I interviewed with one very famous red colored airline, and in those days we were actually weighed! Imagine my hips fitting through the aisles? No way, next! I ended up in the insurance industry when I first came to Canada as my first job, and I simply didn't leave. It wasn't until I hit 41 that I fell into my dream job as The Pink Coach. Being an entrepreneur was so unexpected for me in my life, but has brought about so many blessings it would take another chapter to talk about it all! Imagine. Last year I attended an amazing Robin Sharma event. It was a dream come true and impacted the way I do business and look at my life. We were asked to write our eulogy. What people would say about us once we had died? Wow. Talk about tears. Growing up I had a fear about death, but no more. If tomorrow never comes that's okay, I have lived a full and blessed life, because I live each day like it could be my last. So, follow your dreams! Live life and dream big, the bigger the better! And remember don't worry about what the naysayers tell you about your dreams! You have one chance at this thing called life, there is no dress rehearsal. How many of us live our lives as if it was the last day on earth?

"Today you are You, that is truer than true.
There is no one alive who is You'er than You."
~Dr. Seuss

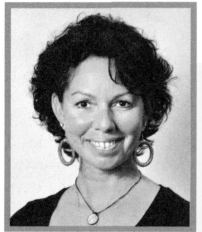

Claudine Pereira is the founder of The Pink Coach, Business Coaching and Consulting. Claudine assists small business owners with fundamental behavioral change. Her consistent and captivating approach stretches her clients to move beyond a limiting sense of self and achieve their desired personal and professional goals. Claudine lives in Toronto with her family and in her spare time can be found dancing or teaching her world class How to Sell like a Beach Vendor program! Contact her at www.thepinkcoach.com

Destiny's Child

The loud explosion reverberated throughout the neighborhood.

The red and orange flame with thick billowing smoke shot out of the open blown out window. There stood the old top loading wooden stove with the cast door handle in the middle of the rental bedroom. The single draft rod now lay on the ground from the explosion.

Blood curdling screams sounded as the hot burning soot had ravaged her tiny 18-month old body. The soot had jetted out ferociously onto the antique white wooden baby crib. Her entire left leg had caught on fire, as her nylon pants melted into her body and onto the mattress. BOOM! It was another deafening explosion, as the fire hurled onto her stomach, burning her baby flesh.

Her mother frantically navigated the thick black smoke to find her baby. Blinded by the soot, she followed the shrill cry of her little girl. She knew nothing of heroism, risking her own life to save her daughter who had been napping alone in her room at the time. After all - she was a mother.

"My daughter is not going to die!" her father; distraught, desperately screamed at the hospital staff.

It was time to take drastic action. The doctors had a new drug that had never before been used to treat children. Close to tasting death, they decided that it was worth the risk. It was a miracle really. She was a fighter. This child was destined to live.

Medicine in the 1960's certainly wasn't what it is today. The doctors had instructed the Mother not to coddle her daughter while she attempted to learn to walk again. The skin graft on the little girls' leg made it difficult to walk. The noticeable scars left both legs looking and feeling completely different from one another. The mother was told that the key to parenting this little girl was Tough Love.

So here I am, Destiny's Child. I am still not sure what my entire purpose is, but I can tell you, my struggles in life have prepared me to share my story of trials and triumph. I can also tell you, that my body, outlook on life and body image were forever changed by that fire.

It wasn't easy growing up having burn scars. Adults and other children viewed me as abnormal. I was often treated as different. They were cruel, to say the least. I truly think that is why I went to food as my savior.

Food became my only friend. It was comfort, non-judgmental, and accepted me as I was and no matter what size I was or what I looked like. I morphed into being an obese child. That had its own challenges, mentally and physically.

At a young age, I was put on all sorts of diets to help me lose weight, to no "success." In school, I was never awarded the lead roles in the plays we were performing. I was assigned "The MOM", as mother's are plump and cuddly. I have bitter memories of being not just teased but bullied on the school bus. I walked down the aisle to find an empty seat as the older kids would make elephant noises. As soon as I would arrive home, I bolted to my "friend" – My secret stash, located in the barn on our property. Oh, how delicious and inviting were the chips, candy, pop, and the best – the half moon chocolate with white crème. It comforted me as I would cry uncontrollably. I truly thought it was my secret, but what you eat in private, unfortunately shows up in public. My "secret" stash caused me to gain even more weight and led me to feel even more terrible about myself.

Shopping for Plus Size clothes today, is totally different than it was when I was a child. Finding clothes had always been a challenge, and I didn't have many choices. More often than not, it wasn't about style, but rather "wear what fits." I found what fit, but they were boy clothes, overalls and old fashioned clothes. I remember going shopping one day and I saw these shirts with houses on them (I remember thinking, 'let's show people that I'm big as a house'), or even with large size animals on them ('I'm big as an animal'). Why do designers think that Plus Size people don't want to look nice when we go somewhere?

As someone who has tried so many diets, as well as support groups, I can tell you THAT list is LONG. To me, the word DIET symbolized something temporary. Eat healthy, lose weight then STOP, then START again. This never seemed to work for me. I realize now, that I just wanted to fit in and be the same as other people. That was was not my destiny.

I had developed severe depression; I exhibited cutting behavior, and even tried to commit suicide. Other illnesses developed due to my obesity: High blood pressure, Type 2 Diabetes, lack of balance and falling. In hindsight, I can't believe how much my life was focused on my size and what that had done to me.

Fat shaming is everywhere.

It has been my experience, that being Plus Size, people view us differently.

We are often looked down upon by others - especially when it comes to finding love, dating and having a family.

Friends mean well, and I had been set up on blind dates. Although they had the best intentions, well, let us just say, that they were so horrible. One particular time, a man took me to a bar, went to get drink - and he never came back. Dumped, I sat there stunned and ashamed, while trying to figure out what do to next. After many attempts to find love, I finally signed up to a well-known dating site.

I started chatting with this younger guy named Bradley. He was also a plump person, he was interested in me, and he wanted to go out. I wasn't sure about him, as there was a very big age difference. Bradley happened to be 10 years younger. So, out of my comfort zone - I decided to go on that date. That date truly changed my life!

Bradley and I have been married for 10 years, together for 15 and we still have a wonderful relationship to this day. It truly makes my life awesome. We were not lucky enough to have children (because of my health issues), but we do have fur babies and other family.

June 2014 WAS DECISION TIME!

I decided that I was going to get healthier as I now weighed 353 pounds. The dreaded 400 pounds wasn't too far away. This weight was my breaking point. I was having difficulty doing everyday activities like walking or putting on my shoes. I was determined to get on track. I found a product that became an absolute life saver for me. I started to lose weight, slowly building my confidence. I felt so good about myself and was able to move my body! I noticed that a brand new gym was being built and I was determined to join. In February, Bradley and I signed up before it was completely built.

Then in March I started getting very bad headaches. It felt like I had a woodpecker in my head and the pain proceeded to get worse and worse. My doctor sent me for tests, I remember a sick feeling in the pit of my stomach as I waited anxiously to find out the results. Then, on March 20, those results came and they hit me like a ton of bricks.

"Petra, you have swelling on your brain, an infection of the brain, and a tumor the size of half a mandarin orange."

I immediately went into shock. The doctor continued, "Go to the hospital right now. They are waiting for you."

I had officially been thrown a curve ball. On March 24, I had brain surgery to remove the tumor. I was relieved when the doctors told me that I did not have cancer. Four days later, on March 28, I was discharged from the hospital and I went home to recover.

I spent three months at home recovering from surgery, and then, at the end of June, the gym that Bradley and I joined opened its doors. On the club scales during my first visit, I weighed in at 337 lbs. First on the agenda... working out with Team Burn!

In the beginning, it was challenging to work out as an obese person and at the same time dealing with staples in my head from the surgery. On one of those days I had been working out, I looked around and felt like I was the biggest person there. I just couldn't do as many of the exercises as the others, and I ran out crying.

One of the instructors caught me before I left and told me that it wasn't that I couldn't do it, it was just that I wasn't allowed to do those moves yet. We came up with a strategy that when I wasn't able or allowed to perform a certain exercise, I would just say "let's modify" and I was given a different exercise.

To date, I feel like a brand new ME. I feel so confident and energized.

So far, I have lost 60 pounds, with a total of 77 inches. I am off 8 medications and have been off insulin for a year. Many people want to know how I have gotten to this point. I have shared with them as I am sharing with you, that it has definitely a journey. My mindset has completely changed. I have consciously worked on my health, body, beauty, and confidence all at the same time as you can't just change one part and think the weight will stay off. Once you decide that you want to make a change, it is important that you work on all of the aspects of your life.

My biggest tip: never cut out eating anything from your food plan. Do not deprive yourself. As soon as you say to yourself that you can't have something like chips or chocolate, that is the moment that you set yourself up for a set back–and even worse, spiraling back to the habits that you had before. You don't want to feel that you have sabotaged your "diet." Have it, enjoy it, so that you aren't constantly thinking of wanting the "bad" things and you take a bite and you have now ruined it.

Today, I cook, shop, and work out differently. Most of all, I am determined to keep myself mentally healthy because having depression can cause some major obstacles in your life. The biggest part of doing this, I have found, is being around positive people, going to the club, and working with different trainers - because they all teach me something different. I keep myself busy too. I just love taking different classes like painting, going to movies with my incredibly supportive husband, hanging with friends, volunteering, and even doing things by myself.

Clothes shopping is now enjoyable! I buy clothes that I love to wear (the louder the better!) and that make me feel good. Whenever I have the opportunity, I help others at the gym as I know what it feels like to be a big person working out at the club and feeling like I don't belong. I do on occasion have members come up to me and say that they are glad that there are Plus Size people at the gym. The old me, would have freaked out on them. Today, I am still Plus Size and I love myself. I enjoy showing them my before picture and share my story as it has been posted at the club.

I do realize that I am a work in progress.

I continue to strive and succeed in my healthier journey. I was born that fighter! That Destiny's Child. I embrace the goal to lose more weight. After all, I have much more life to live, more crazy outfits to wear, and I have to remove more medications from my life.

It certainly is not easy, but I can tell you, with all the confidence in the world, I am so worth it!

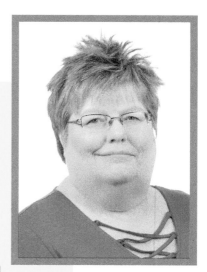

Petra Reiss Wilson was born in Germany in 1964, and moved to Toronto with her family in 1970. She completed a certificate program in research based writing at George Brown College in 1995. Currently Petra volunteers with Team Chelsea Animal Rescue in Durham Region where she lives with her husband Bradley and her two cats Rusty, Nicki and one dog named Lindsay. She keeps things positive in her life and works on her bucket list.

Sarah Shakespeare

Starting and Finishing the Story Together

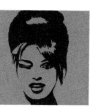

Growing up in England in the 70's was a lot of fun, especially when it was in a Jamaican household. My mother was English and my dad was Jamaican. They met each other 5 weeks after my dad moved to England in 1965. My mom was a 17-year -old white English girl, and my dad a Jamaican man aged 32. To say that they didn't have the approval of my mother's family at first is an undestatement! So it took a while for my dad to gain acceptance from his in-laws, but since he was a happy, friendly man he soon became part of the family. My mother spent most of her time with my dad and they were inseparable right from the beginning.

They were a social couple and people soon realized that they were destined to 'be'. My dad was a lot of fun and loved parties and meeting people, and so did my mother, so it was a fun relationship from the start. And so the amazing story of Trescott and Christine began.

They continued the fun life for many years and had their first child, my brother, Philip in 1972. My dad left the hospital after his birth in a bad mood because he was 'so white', and had not expected his son to have such light colored skin! My mother soon calmed him down the next day as she explained to him what a 'mixed race' child looked like. I was born eleven months later with his full approval since he was prepared for my fairer color ahead of time! They moved into their permanent family home when I was two months old in December of 1973. My sister Rachel came as a welcomed addition to the family in 1984, when I was ten years old.

We were a full, happy family. My dad was a big church-goer and we went to church each week. My mother didn't attend church regularly and would spend time at home cooking and cleaning while we were out. We, of course were always welcomed home afterwards by the smell of a lovely Sunday dinner! It wasn't the smell of an English traditional roast dinner; it was the smell of a traditional Jamaican meal. My mother, although born and raised in England had adopted many of my father's Jamaican traditions into our family life. We were very used to the smell of 'Jerk Chicken and Rice' in our household.

I met my husband Paul when I was only 16 years old and immediately fell in love. We had our first daughter, Abigail, two years later. When I was 26 years old we moved to Canada, and although I had a wonderful family, great friends and an amazing job, I still listened to my inner voice and followed my instincts and emigrated. I settled into my life in Canada easily, but still talked to my parents twice a day. Two years after moving to Canada I had my second daughter, Hannah. Now there was a real incentive to get back to England for more family holidays with, yet another, grandchild!

I was expecting my third child when I received a phone call from my mother. She told me that my dad had been taken into hospital. He was so sick that his organs were shutting down. And he had been asking for me. The doctors had also indicated that family and good friends should come to make a final visit. In that moment I questioned my move to Canada. I told my mother that I would be there as soon as I could. And I told her to ask him to wait for me.

I had been told by my dad since I was a young girl that I would be the 'last pretty little face' that he would see when he died. I felt like I had to keep up my part of the deal and be there at the end. I booked an emergency appointment with my doctor for a note to show the airline to allow me to travel. I wasn't far away from my due date. My doctor recommended that I didn't fly, and said that it would pose a risk to the baby. I insisted. I had a deal with my dad that I would not break. I would be the last face that he saw when he passed away. He performed more tests, and reluctantly wrote me a note to travel. He insisted that I be back 6 weeks before the baby's due date as the airline may not let me board the plan to come back to Canada. I felt like it was a risk that I was prepared to make so that I could see my father for the last time.

Although I was married with children, I had always called my dad my greatest love of my life. I wasn't ready to say goodbye, but knew that he was expecting me. I called my brother, Philip, once I had everything arranged, and told him that I was on the way. I told him to tell my dad to wait for me. The flight felt longer than the usual nine hours and I was restless and anxious the whole time, worried that I wouldn't make it in time. I had to be the last pretty little face he saw.

I landed, only to endure a two hour drive to the hospital. I called my dad's hospital room and received no answer, but I tried not to think the worst. I had lived my whole life with a positive mindset, so I refused to think thathe hadn't waited for me. When I walked into his room his bed was surrounded by my family and close friends. My mother, at his bedside whispered to my dad, "She's here." I walked over and smiled and said, "Thank you for waiting for me."

He couldn't talk as he was so heavily medicated and weak. I sat down, held his hand, and started the first, of what would be our normal, daily conversations. The next day, he remained the same, but the day after that he showed slight improvement, and they had lessened his pain medication. The news was out that dad was leaving us so we had many visitors. One of my dad's very close friends came to visit, and when he saw me at the bedside he said, "I don't have to say goodbye to him now because you're here. You are his Angel and this isn't the end." He kissed my cheek, thanked me for coming, and left.

My dad's health started to improve by the third day of me arriving. I sat by his bedside all day, every day. He continued to improve over the days and I felt like I had just witnessed a miracle. He was home from the hospital in three weeks in good health, and it was time for me to get back to Canada to welcome the new baby, Emily Jane, and see her sisters, and her dad. Trescott had decided he wasn't ready to go just yet.

Three years later got a surprise call from my mother. It was about 7:00 a.m. and I was used to her calling at 8:30 a.m. She immediately said, "Well, I've got it," to which I answered, "Got what?" "You know, they found 'it' at my test last week. I have to have a mastectomy." I knew that she had been for a mammogram a couple of weeks before, but since we hadn't talked about it again I had thought that it was just a routine appointment. It took a few seconds to take it in, and as I could feel myself starting to feel dizzy as I realized what 'it' was. I told my mother that I would call her back in five minutes. I layed on my bed and stared at the ceiling. How had this happened? I took my five minutes to take this all in, and then promptly called my mother back. A lump had been found in her breast and it was cancerous. We talked about her otions. The doctor wanted to go for a mastectomy, and it was scheduled in 2 weeks.

Once again the life we built in Canada seemed ill-planned. I knew in that instant that I had to leave and go back to England to look after her. I had a husband, 3 daughters, and was building a new house. I told her that I would there when she came home from her operation and made my plans to leave Canada. I tried to stay positive about the outcome. My three daughters were then aged two, seven, and seventeen. I had a busy husband who worked more than full time with his business. I decided the best plan was to take the youngest, Emily Jane, with me, and leave Abigail and Hannah with their dad.

It was a hard two weeks as I prepared to leave while keeping up, of course, with my daily phone calls. Neither of my parents had their usual enthusiastic, happy energy when I called. They were both very pleased when I said that I would be coming back to England until further notice. I arrived on the day of her surgery. It allowed me to spend time with my father, explaining the procedure, and reassuring him we would have her home soon. I arrived at the hospital to find my mother looking very ill, and weak. She was, however, very happy to see me.

So the days of recovery started in the hospital. I would visit mom all day and into the evening. My mother-in-law lived locally, and happily agreed to watch Emily Jane each day so that I could visit my mother at the hospital, and help my father at home. Good friends of the family set up a schedule to look after my father while I was with my mom. Rachel and Philip would also help where needed. They too, had to digest this news about our mother, and deal with the uncertainty of what the future held.

As the first week passed, she still felt extremely tired. The doctors were concerned she wasn't healing very well, so she was sent for more tests. This test was for a scan of her back, and was scheduled at another hospital. I wasn't allowed to travel in the ambulance with her so I traveled separately. As I entered the scan department, I saw a lady waiting to check in, patiently sitting in a wheelchair. It took me a minute to realize it was my mother.For the first time since I had arrived in England, I saw her as a woman with cancer. She looked up and smiled, and I tried not to cry.

The sadness overcame me and my body started to ache. I was already suspicious that my mother's cancer had spread because I had given her a back and shoulder massage the day before and I could feel lump after lump in her upper back. They were not there before, and here we were to have a back scan. I knew that if I could feel the lumps then the machine would definitely see them. I was right. The cancer had spread. In a conversation with a cancer specialist it was decided that chemotherapy would be more painful than the pain she was already enduring. And it would not guarantee a longer life.

The cancer had spread so much she was now classed as terminally ill. I cried right in front of the doctor as we talked through the diagnosis. We were already talking about controlling her pain with heavy drugs to make her more comfortable, and using words like palliative care. This was so hard to hear when I was expecting to be caring for her back home, helping her heal after her surgery. Now it was time for me to tell her. I walked to her room and she simply said, "So it's not good news, then?" I said "How do you know?" She told me I might want to look in a mirror because my makeup was smudged all over my face, and that I looked like a character from the 'Rocky Horror Picture Show'. "You would only cry if it was bad news." She was right. I relayed back to her exactly what the doctor had said to me and we just sat there quietly. Within a few minutes my mother's lifetime friend Gladys appeared. Her timing couldn't have been any better.

They had been friends for 45 years and my mother needed her friend at that very minute. I told Gladys the news, and left them to sit and chat. It was now an afternoon of phone calls for me as I informed family and friends that, indeed, we were going to be saying goodbye to our lovely lady in the next 4-6 months. I drove to my parents' house and sat with my father and told him the news. This was, perhaps, harder than telling my mom. His face was the saddest thing that I would ever seen. We had tried to live in hope that everything was going to be okay, but today we had been told it wasn't going to be. I spent the rest of the afternoon with dad, and he wanted the evening to phone their personal friends to tell them of the news. I was back to the hospital to see my mother by the evening and we carried on the evening peacefully.

I began reading a book every night about stages of cancer. I would read about 'months before death', 'weeks before death', 'days before death', and 'hours before death'. I wanted to be truly informed about what to expect. I brought her favorite foods to her every day as the hospital food was not very appetizing! I was asked about hospice care and rest home care. I declined both and insisted she would go home to the house that she had lived in for 36 years to spend her final weeks there. It was a definite struggle to persuade the hospital to agree with my request because she would need medical attention throughout the day. After many lengthy meetings I managed to get her home with a full room set up on the ground level with a hospital bed, oxygen, and nurses scheduled to care for her every four hours thought the day and night. It was time to get her home.

It was the middle of May, so I arranged for my other daughters to come from Canada at the end of June when school was out. But suddenly her symptoms and behaviors that meant 'months/weeks before death' changed to 'days before death'. I always trust my instincts. I was glad I had read about the cancer stages, and called Paul immediately to ask him to come straightaway. He booked the flights and arrived with Abigail and Hannah the next day. It was Saturday. She wasn't communicating very well but could still string a few words together. Lots of people came to the house to see her over the weekend. On Monday one of the nurses said to me, "Your mother needs to relax now. She is close to the end, and we need her to relax and let go."

I knew exactly what to do. She loved music so I arranged a 'farewell' just for family and close friends. We played all of her favorite music and sang along. She had stopped communicating at this point, and was on the highest dose of Morphine to make her comfortable. We took turns holding her hands, and we danced and sang, knowing that she was smiling so big on the inside. I know she felt the love from her three children as we sang and danced to songs that she had taught us in our childhood. The party carried on until 2:00 a.m. without one complaint from the neighbors; they knew that it was Christine's final hours.

She was peaceful, and I got my father to sit with her for the morning. He agreed that she would have loved her Reggae music farewell party. At noon she was relaxed enough to take her last breath, with her family at her side. Although you know it's coming, nothing can prepare you for the pain you feel when the heart stops. It's final; it's sad, and your whole body is numb. I didn't think that my dad's face could be any sadder than it had already been; today was his saddest day.

Many people came to the house pay their respects, she had been a very popular woman and it showed with the many messages of condolences that I received.

I then started to plan the Celebration of Life. I had an absolute vision of what it would look like, and it was the perfect day. We had a 12 page color booklet made about her life as a keepsake for guests to take with them. I wanted her to have a send-off like a Queen. I booked limousines for the friends and family, ordered beautiful flowers, and, of course, some of her favorite songs for the church service. It was hard day for us all on the day of the funeral, but my dad took it very hard. He was weak and tired, and it took all of his will just to get into the car to go the church. He had a wheelchair all day because he was too weak to stand. He had been to the Chapel of Rest every day to sit with her for many hours. He wasn't ready after 45 years to say goodbye.

"There must be an Angel" by The Eurythmics played when she was brought into the church, and music filled the service, and the whole day. The church was full as 350 people made the effort to attend that day. She was a very popular lady and loved by many. We continued to sing songs at the graveside as we filled in the hole and mounted it with a sea of flowers. The party afterwards saw guests dancing and singing from a complete playlist of her favorite songs. We had a wonderful Jamaican caterer, who impressed many of the Jamaican guests! We ended the celebration with lots of lovely coconut cake to eat at midnight. It was actually the perfect day, and she would have loved every minute of it.

When I took my father home and helped him get ready for bed he said to me, "What use is it for me to go on now?" Just two weeks after her funeral my dad had a most unusual day. My dad liked a good funeral and raised us to believe that funerals were a very important way to pay our respects when a person left us. There had been many of late; it seemed that he was attending a funeral every Friday! There was a funeral of a friend that day, but he said that he wasn't going today. If only there had been a book on 'Dying of a Broken Heart' I would have known that was a sign from the chapter 'hours before death'. There were several signs that day, but I missed them all.

166

Sign #1 – missing a funeral.

Sign #2 – My dad was famous for his tea drinking; he only drank a half cup of tea all day.

Sign #3 – I had a family friend that was due to call in on him at night to check that he was OK. He insisted I stay with him.

Sign #4 – He always took his panic button everywhere he went, always hanging it around his neck. He left it on his cupboard downstairs that night.

During the evening we locked eyes for about 15 seconds, neither of us saying anything. I think that he was saying, "What is this girl going to do without me?" Before he settled down for the evening he felt hot, and was dizzy. I called the doctor in. She came and checked him out, with pads and wires all over to check his heart. She said he was fine and off she went. I confirmed with my dad just a few minutes later that the doctor said he had "check out fine". He asked me, "Which doctor?" That was **Sign #5**.

We chatted and laughed and hugged, and I went downstairs to tidy the living room as I knew that we would have visitors the next day. I nodded off, exhausted, in a chair, and was jolted awake a few minutes later short of breath and with a pounding heart. I stood and went upstairs to find my father, the love of my life, had left me. It was just like the plan had always been, I was the 'last pretty little face' that he saw before he went back home. I just stood there in his blue pajamas crying and wishing that it wasn't true.

I had five signs that day, but didn't realize that they were telling me this was his last day. It was the worst moment of my life, standing there, helpless. A pain like I had never felt before ran through my body, engulfed by grief and sadness. I was told that he died from heart failure in less than 11 seconds. I was out of breath with a pounding heart for probably about 11 seconds. That had been our final connection.

I called an ambulance, but could hardly speak through the sobs. I was numb and weak. He was a ready gone by the time the ambulance arrived but, I knew that. It was exactly two weeks after my mother's funeral. Hadn't he said, "Tip me now, I'm ready," and, "What use is it that I go on now?" My life had changed drastically over a space of just four weeks. The two most influential people in my life had left me. And I was about to plan another Celebration of Life, and did we have a lot to celebrate about this amazing man!

In my grief I stayed focused and positive. I took one day at a time, and worked towards the day two weeks away. A full 16 page memory book of his life was made for the guests to take away. A horse and carriage was booked as a symbolic Jamaican tradition to take you 'home'. It was decorated with flowers and the horses wore the Jamaican colors on their bridals. Limousines took the guests to the church behind the horse and carriage. As we approached the church, my heart swelled to witness a sea of people in the street. The church could not hold the 500 people at his funeral. It wasn't just me that thought he was an amazing man!

The song "Day-O" by Harry Belafonte welcomed him into the church. We included beautiful hymns that I knew were his favorites. But we also had "Hot, Hot, Hot" by Arrow during the middle of the Service, which certainly got people tapping their feet. I stood by his casket to pay my respects as 'our' song was played, Celine Dion, "Because You Loved Me". As he left the church we heard, "Jamaican Farewell". He was reunited with Christine in the same burial plot. I was still in shock and denial that this had even happened, and found myself reading the plaque on his coffin many times to confirm it was really him. The party afterwards was, again, amazing, and many people shared personal stories of both him and Christine. This time is was carrot cake at midnight!

Many called it the 'end of an era'. Trescott and Christine were a popular couple, and they were going to be sadly missed. I truly believe he died from a broken heart. They may not have been the perfect couple, but they were the perfect parents for me. On the day of my father's service a friend said to me, "Sarah, he started his journey with your mother, and now he's meeting her to go and finish up the journey together. It's their story from start to finish. You are part of the story, but you have your own story. Keep living your story."

So I keep living my story as they would want me to. They taught me to be happy, positive and enthusiastic. So I am just that, and living life to the fullest, just as they would expect of me. This loss of my parents in a short space of time has taught me many things. Life is an absolute gift; treat it that way. Love your family, and let them know it; distance is no excuse, as I have proven. Live your life to the fullest, and do things that make you laugh right down to your feet! Although we are devastated by their passing, we must celebrate the amazing people that have influenced us in our life. Make it your business to know what type of celebration your family members want before they leave us.

Trescott and Christine are buried together and have a beautiful headstone that the family fondly calls the 'monument'. On my visits to England, and my hometown, my first stop is at the cemetery. They would like that nothing has changed, and that I drive from the airport straight to my 'parents', just like I always did before.

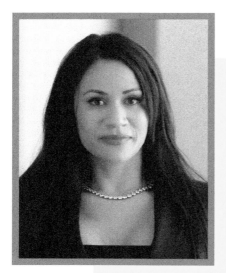

Sarah Shakespeare has always lived her with a "Glass is Full" attitude. As a Personal Trainer and Coach for near- ly 25 years she loves to help people enrich their life through creating a healthy lifestyle. As someone who is very goal driven, she has come to know that success really comes from first sculpting a positive mindset. She is a wife, mother of three daughters was born and raised in England. She lives in beautiful British Columbia, Canada and feels lucky everyday to live in her dream destination!

Gillian Joy Whyatt

Daddy: I was always his Angel and now he's mine

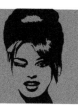

The day my daddy died, my entire world changed.

It's the phone call you never want to get, especially if you live in another province. So far away. Takes planning and resources to get you to where you need to go.

Sooner or later, we all get this call.

My mom took my dad to the hospital because he wasn't feeling well, stomach upset then pain in his chest.

Until that day, my dad was pretty darn healthy for a man of 69. He was in the hospital for kidney stones years before, and this other time when he had 3rd degree burns on his arm from a job.

They admitted my dad, and urgently airlifted him to another hospital when they discovered blockages. He died five days later.

Within that short stay at the hospital he had a stroke (possibly more than one) and two more heart attacks. My dad died of a massive heart attack.

He was unable to speak due to the stroke so he used a whiteboard to communicate. Before he died, he wrote "massive heart attack" on the whiteboard. He also said his pain was a 10 ++++. Those were his last words.

That was not supposed to happen. I wasn't ready to let him go! I fell apart!

When I got the call, I left my husband and 3 daughters in a rush. My brother and I left right away on a flight to see my dad, who had since suffered a stroke after a surgical procedure.

That flight was the longest flight I've ever been on. I felt helpless, agitated and scared. Being disconnected from the world, not knowing what news I would hear when I arrived— was he still with us, would I get to hug him again and feel his strong arms around me and soft beard on my cheek? My heart raced with these thoughts. When I thought of him laying there, I could feel his pain. I was scared and I knew he was too.

When I got to see my dad, he couldn't speak to me because the stroke had left him partially paralyzed. I saw and felt the love in his eyes as he saw me come into the room. He lit up. He was so happy to see me.

He lifted his arms the best he could to create a heart with his hands and then he reached for me, taking me into his still strong arms that had held me and cared for me my entire life.

He very much still had his wits about him. I was able to see from his expressions he was frustrated.

It broke my heart seeing him there in that hospital bed, so helpless. My dad hadn't been helpless a day in his life. He always came to the rescue of others, not the other way around. He was desperate to heal from the stroke so they would do the bypass.

My dad did everything the nurses instructed him to do. He didn't want to be there, he was on the mend.

We had 2 days with my dad. We chatted with him. We held his hand. We helped him use a whiteboard to communicate. We kept his mouth moist because he couldn't swallow or move his tongue, which he kept biting. I would have done anything for him. I know he would have done the same for me. That's what we did in our family. We took care of each other no matter what.

The day he died, we were tired. We'd spent every moment we could by his side. He motioned to us that he was fine and practically pushed us out the door.

We told him we loved him. Then my brother, my mom and I went out to get a breath of fresh air, some food and a few things dad would need.

My mom's phone rang. It was her friends. They were frantic. They told us to get back to the hospital as soon as possible.

But it was too late. The doctors were working on my dad, giving him chest compressions. I could barely see. He was lying there helpless.

This wasn't supposed to happen. He was getting better, not worse.

My mind was racing. I was going crazy. I felt like I was going to faint.

This can't be happening. It can't. Can I really be losing my dad?

Don't tell me my worst nightmare is coming true.

The nurses sat us all down in a nearby empty room. We started to sob.

We knew what was happening. We were losing our hero. Our best friend. The man who loved everyone. He had a heart of gold and would do absolutely anything for anyone.

The doctors came to tell us he was gone. I collapsed.

My mom and my brother came to me and we held on tight.

I didn't recognize the sounds that came from inside me. I emitted a sound of such despair, a sound that hurt and broke my heart and the pain I felt deep in my bones.

The sound that came from me was foreign, coming from a pain unlike no other I've ever felt before. It was raw and deep and I was lost. Our lives had changed irrevocably in an instant. The physical bond between my dad and myself was severed.

My dad had left the earth. I felt myself breaking. I felt such pain, such grief, such loss.

I felt numb and heavy, like the weight of the world had just come crashing down on me. I couldn't breathe. I couldn't catch my breath between the sobs.

A piece of me died along with him that evening in December.

Just two weeks before Christmas, my daddy was really gone. I didn't want happy, good feeling Christmas around me. It didn't match how I was feeling. When I returned I was numb. I felt nothing, besides the pain of losing my daddy. I wanted to be happy for my daughters and husband. I fought to enjoy Christmas. All presents were bought online that year and delivered to my home. I couldn't even step into a bustling shopping mall surrounded by the Christmas lights, colors and music that I normally loved. The memories of Christmas past with both my mom and dad flashing in my mind. I would no longer get to hear his voice sing to me on the phone or wish me a Merry Christmas. I was devastated.

He wasn't just away on some extended business trip this time, or vacationing with my beautiful mom. No, this time, he was gone.

Gone forever.

He touched so many lives. Grown men cried when they heard of my father's passing. He was an angel on earth to many people.

Grief overtook me as I went through the motions of everyday life. A dark fog enveloped me and followed me everywhere. I was no longer the same woman I had been when I arrived at the hospital. Now I was a woman, mother and wife without my dad by my side, to cheer me on in difficult times, no phone calls with a joke, story or a song.

He always knew how to make me laugh no matter how I was feeling. He knew how to work his magic and lift the fog and the clouds when life got hard. Now what was I supposed to do? The fog and clouds settled into my life and he wasn't there to rescue me or lift me out of the dark. He was a bright light in my life. He was a problem solver, a fixer and my life coach.

The day he died, the light in me extinguished.

We all need a mentor. Be it a parent or a friend or a business mentor. It's important to surround yourself with people who lift you up and cheer you on, support you and guide you. Life doesn't come with Instructions. We were not created to live life alone and or figure things out on our own. We need to learn from others who have learned and made mistakes along the way.

I would soon meet my mentors and friends who would help me in my journey.

When I got back home, my family didn't know what to do or say. We cried and mourned in our own ways. I took time off work and found myself sobbing uncontrollably all of a sudden, without warning. The grief was so deep, the pain so strong that it overtook my life. So many times I wanted to call him, to ask a question, to get his advice.

And then one day I realized that if my dad were here he would be saying:

"Missy, come on let's go, we've got work to do, nothing's going to get done if you stay in the dumps, cheer up and let's make it happen!"

It was time.

For years I struggled. Life always seemed to be one struggle after another. I learned to constantly be solving problems, and or creating them as that's all I knew. I recognized that the choices I made had me stuck in a constant state of problems and struggle.

My mom and dad were always by my side. Regardless of what province they lived in. They were always there.

My dad had a gypsy heart and that gypsy resides in me as well. He loved to travel, experience new things and seek adventure.

I decided I would make my dad proud. I would no longer struggle and wait for things to happen. I would make life happen for me, not to me!

I was ready for my journey to begin. The adventure of a lifetime was waiting for me.

I didn't really have a plan. I had a mindset that I was done struggling, that I would do something with my life so my family could have more time with me. We would spend more time together. Travel. Time is something we never get back. I began to manifest my life.

> "Grief is like the ocean; it comes in waves,
> ebbing and flowing. Sometimes the water
> is calm, and sometimes it is overwhelming.
> All we can do is learn to swim."
> ~Vicki Harrison

I was ready to be the Captain of my own ship on the Sea of Life. Sailing towards a new discovery. Course correcting along the way, to find my inner peace. My new life. The life I chose to create. During the storms, my dad continued to be the Lighthouse, which helped me find my way.

We can let grief take our lives over. We can allow it to swallow us up but that's not living. Would your loved ones want that for you? I began thinking about this and realized that if my dad was here in physical form he would encourage me and lift me up. He would tell me to live my life and make it the best.

> "Grief, I've learned, is really love. It's all the love you want to give but cannot give. The more you loved someone, the more you grieve. All of that unspent love gathers up in the corners of your eyes and in that part of your chest that gets empty and hollow feeling. The happiness of love turns to sadness when unspent. Grief is just love with no place to go."
> ~Jamie Anderson

I attended a Leadership Empowerment workshop Mother's Day weekend. It changed my life. I finally had a plan. I met some amazing mentors and felt my dad's presence the entire time.

I knew he would be so jazzed and excited about what I was learning.

Something awakened and opened up within me that weekend. The light began to shine again. And so did I. I found myself again – the Joy that was lost for so long.
I learned that focus determines behavior and behavior determines results. So it was time to focus.

I decided to make it happen. I continued to learn these skills. I wanted to equip myself to live the best life that I could.

I wanted to make my dad proud. Although he was no longer physically here with me I realized that he will always be in my heart and memories.

I can hear his words of encouragement in my mind, because he spoke them my entire life. What a gift that I'm able to recall his voice and his words whenever I want.

During this time I learned the power of the unconscious mind and the Mind/Body connection. It's such a fascinating subject to study.

Since my teenage years I've been a lucid dreamer. As an adult I began to have fewer lucid dreams.

My dad was always a lucid dreamer as well. We both have active imaginations. Our unconscious minds go haywire when we sleep. We woke up telling the craziest dreams to those around us and they would be entertained by what we shared. We were always similar and connected in more ways than one.

> "A lucid dream is a dream during which the dreamer is aware of dreaming. During lucid dreaming, the dreamer may be able to exert some degree of control over the dream characters, narrative, and environment."
> ~https://en.wikipedia.org/wiki/Lucid_dream

One night my dad was in my thoughts a lot. I was picturing having a conversation with him about my journey and what I've been learning. I then out loud said "I wish I could just give you a hug and tell you I love you."

That night I had a lucid dream! I was in a room full of people, just chatting and mingling. I look across the room and I say to myself "Hey, that's dad, but he's gone and— omigosh I must be dreaming because he's no longer with us." I knew this was my opportunity to go over to him to get that hug and tell him that I love him. When I began to cross the room, he saw me and smiled that big awesome smile and his eyes lit up. I went straight into his arms and held him tight! Feeling his beard tickle my cheek, I even smelled cigarette smoke slightly and I said "Daddy, I love you so much." I held on tight for as long as I could knowing that I was dreaming. I woke up smiling.

What a gift! This gave me hope.

What is the difference now that he's no longer physically here with me? He's always in my memories, the sound of his voice, and the twinkle of his shining eyes when he smiled. These memories are forever with me. Because I am a part of him and he is a part of me. This gave me hope. I didn't lose my dad. He lives within me. I'm continuing his work, touching lives and bringing awareness to others about their infinite potential.
I was ecstatic.

After this Leadership Empowerment weekend I attended, I realized that I needed to learn more for myself and the transformation I needed to go through. I also realized that this was the work I was meant to do using what I learned. I began doing some intense personal breakthroughs using Neuro Linguistic Programming and Hypnosis. I began to understand the power of the unconscious mind. I began to understand that we are the ones who make the decisions about how we think and feel; we need to reprogram, rewire and change our thinking. It's all about choice and I choose Happy, Healthy and Wealthy.

"Missy, you always have a choice, you can be and or do anything you want to".

I finally began to understand what my very wise daddy was telling me. He mentored and coached me my entire life. He taught me about life and encouraged me to look at the brighter side. To see someone else's perspective. He taught me empathy, and because of our gypsy-like lifestyle I learned to enjoy meeting new people. I made new friends wherever I went and met some amazing people.

My dad taught me a lot. He was a natural teacher of life. He continued teaching and sharing with me after he was gone. He still guided me on my path. Every step of the way.

He guided me to seek answers and to journey on. I listened to my heart, my gut, my intuition and I let it lead me and guide me. I didn't do it for anyone else. I became selfish in the pursuit of my purpose and who I was to become.

I was journeying to find 'Joy' once more as she was lost for some time. She was hidden and she was living inside a shell. It was time to grow into the woman that he would be proud of. He was always proud, and now I was going to make myself proud. I was on a mission.

The day my daddy died, he gave me a gift: He left me with the burning desire to make something of my life, to make life count, to enjoy every moment and not to waste a second of it. Because we never know when life will change – or end.

Life is precious! Life is darn right absolutely amazing! Would I do anything to have my dad back in physical form, you betcha, but I've learned to see the beauty in death. He created me with my beautiful mom 42 years ago. The day he died I was reborn.

He gave me life again.

Has life been without its challenges and or struggles since, heck no! And I've looked at each struggle differently. I was conditioned for so many years to learn how to navigate and adjust during hard times. My focus was on the struggle, so that's what was showing up in my life.

I've learned to have a different perspective in regards to hard times etc. I'm looking for the lessons to be learned and how to do things differently going forward.

I've learned to embrace challenges, to feel the fear and do it anyway. To say yes to opportunities and figure it out afterwards. I'm a work in progress. I'm loving this journey of life and I owe it all to my mom and dad for giving me life.

Each year on my birthday I celebrate them: because without them I wouldn't get to experience the joys, the love and the beauty that life provides.

My journey continues. I have learned that life is about living, making choices and not living in the past but learning from it.

Life is not perfect. We all have different beliefs, needs, desires, wants and wishes; and we deserve what our heart desires. We deserve to journey on to discover who we are as women, as mothers, as incredible beings that continue to grow. We're a part of something pretty darn incredible on this miraculous earth.

Now I get to work with people who are struggling and lost in their pain. Some are stuck. Some feel trapped and don't know how to change the circumstances in which they find themselves.

Now I get to give back and that gives me hope. Hope, the power of belief, focus and mindset are what you need to catapult yourself forward.

If you have lost a parent, be kind to yourself. It's ok to rage, cry and grieve but don't stay there too long. You have amazing things to do. Time is something we never get back, and we always feel it slipping by. Make it count, and make it awesome.

I wonder if you are aware of the potential you have within. You were born magnificent. No matter where you are today. You have the ability to be, do or have whatever your heart desires. You may have already started to become aware of your infinite potential. Seek it and achieve it.

These words are dedicated to all dads and the women and daughters who love them.

Not every daughter is as blessed as I am. For those who don't have that same relationship I had, know that you are loved.

That you are the writer of your story. Make it a good one.

> "I will never forget the moment your heart stopped and mine kept beating."
> ~Angela Miller

I love you Daddy!

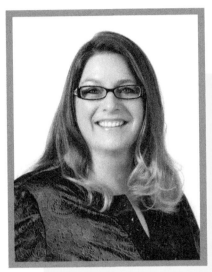

Gillian Joy Whyatt is a Brain Changer, she is a tour guide for your unconscious mind to assist you on the journey and to live your best life! She has always been fascinated by human behavior, psychology and over the last few decades has researched and taken training courses so that she can now live the dream of helping others achieve their dreams.

She's a Master Practitioner of Neuro Linguistic Programming, Time Line Therapy, NLP Coach and Trainer of Hypnosis.

Adriane Breese Lloyd

The Wind Beneath my Wings; Surviving the loss of my identical twin!

It is 5:15 a.m., I am at the hospital, CAMH; the Center for Addictions and Mental Health in the Emergency Assessment Unit (EAU). A year ago, today, I waited for the dreaded, yet anticipated call from the coroner. Exactly to the day, as they said it would be; three months after your death. I was finally going to find out how you passed away and left this world suddenly...

My name is Adriane and I am an alcoholic. I am here to share my experience, strength and hope with you; what it was like, what happened and how is life today.

Immersed in amniotic fluid, floating, so warm and intertwined as one. A knowing soul connection that was cemented in the womb, as well as our shared birth experience. A field of connectedness like no other, a complete consciousness flowing through the amniotic sac. An experience we felt then and which grew throughout childhood.

Identical twins form their identity in the womb especially mono twins; inseminated by one sperm to one egg, divided and became two. Two human beings with the same DNA, everything identical except for our fingerprints. We started our life there together as we held hands and shifted positions

185

never leaving contact with each other; a knowing soul split into two, an experience most people will never experience in their lifetime.

I was born on July 27th, 1962 at 11:20 a.m., and two minutes later (unbeknownst to my mother) my identical twin sister (Baby B as they called her) was born. Diana was breach, in the womb. The Doctor said "there are another set of feet." My mom passed out. We were rushed to the nursery and placed in incubators as we were four weeks premature. Baby "A" was written on my feet and baby "B" on Di's. Diana was larger than I and she got to go home first. This was probably a Godsend for my mother who could then prepare for another baby. Diana was a sickly child and I was the strong one. She would be ill and have febrile seizures.

We met each other's needs socially, emotionally and physically. The result of this was having less interaction with other people. As a twin you don't need other people, you have each other, even a language of your own which I tend to call "twin talk." This has caused me communication problems my entire life. I automatically think that people understand what I am trying to communicate to them while having left out most of the sentence. Di and I could finish each other's sentences and didn't have to say a lot as there was a knowing and understanding like no other. This is sometimes detrimental leaving either twin without a sense of identity or individuality. Our voices were the same. We were always called the "girls" or the "twins" as most people could not tell us apart.

My mother married at a very young age to escape her very abusive, toxic home. She married a tall, dark haired very handsome man who was an Entomologist, an alcoholic – and starkraving mad. He had delusions of grandeur, severe compulsive disorder, and a violent raging temper; not to mention his gambling problem.

Our father was not around much. He worked for a large medical company. He drank, he gambled and he was never home. He was both emotionally and physically unavaiable to the three of us. My mother had no support or help from her biological family. She could not rely on them in any way, nor leave us there for babysitting or care because of the alcoholism. We were so small, only three years old and I have a vivid memory of hiding under an end table in the living room watching blood splattering across the wall while my father was beating my mother. The continued abuse and instability, the alcoholic insanity all took its toll on my mother who became very ill with Sarcoidosis. One day my father left the house saying he was going to get some milk and never returned. My mother was hospitalized and my sister and I were put into foster care. Diana and I were going to stay with "friends" as my mother called them, however they were foster parents.

We were very lucky in that we were never separated. Life would change dramatically and became a living hell. The first home my sister and I went to had another foster child (a boy) as well as their own daughter. At first when my mother saw the house we were to live in she felt comfortable as we had our own room upstairs together. That quickly changed however. Not long after arriving, we were moved to the unfinished basement to a room with two twin beds, a night stand and a cupboard. The other child was put on the other side of the laundry room in the same kind of conditions.

This was not a home. It was a structure of horrors. The woman's husband would come downstairs late at night and sexually abuse first my sister and then I. It was like a Dr. Mengele experiment. I was the stronger twin, I looked after Di and tried to protect her from him. That usually made it worse for me. I never cared as long as he would leave her alone. She was so fragile.

In the evenings after we were sent to bed we could not make any noise or all hell would break loose. We had to be so quiet that we used the drain in the laundry room floor drain as our toilet, so that we didn't have to go upstairs and disturb anyone to use the washroom. If they heard us, he would come downstairs and go on a rampage, beating us and turning into a possessed devil. He always laughed and ridiculed us. I can still hear his evil voice and his laugh and see the sinister look on his face. I thought I knew who Satan was – however this man was the devil in human form.

He would sit me on the counter and tell me that no one would believe us. That we were bad and horrible little creatures who had made our mother sick. She was never coming back to get us and the stories we told would be interpreted as children's make believe or fantasies. There was a knife on the counter, I wanted to put it through him. I didn't know how - he was so big and strong.

We were locked outside some days and ate dog biscuits, grass and green seeds. There were woods nearby and the two of us would go there and play for hours and made our own "Terabithia" a magical imaginary world.

Di and I went to school until grade 3 while living in this house of horrors. Looking back on it now, I realize that the foster parents were also in the throes of alcoholism... another horrendous nightmare as they would yell, scream and fight with one another. The violence was always escalating, especially when alcohol was involved.

I often wondered if there was a God? I would lie in bed at night and have long conversations with Him. Where are you, God? Why have you forsaken us into this life? Was our mother going to live, come back... would she ever rescue us?

Our mother would come and visit when she could. After seeing we had been living in the basement in these horrible conditions she was devastated and lost it. There was a dispute over money. The next day when Di and I came back from our "Terabithia," all of our belongings were on the front lawn.

My new stepfather to be (who will be referred to as my father from here on...) put me on the kitchen counter and looked into my eyes and said tell me what happened here... I hugged him, I couldn't tell him. I thought they would leave us there and not believe us. Diana was crying, lying on the floor at the bottom of the stairs after being thrown down the stairs by the devil. He was laughing, sinister, and denied ever touching her.

My twin and I were placed in two more homes, shortly after. They were "all girl" homes and fortunately they kept us together. Diana and I went to school together, shared the same room, as well as a lot of secrets that we vowed never to reveal. We were so close, a bond like no other.

My mom and dad came and got us and we started living together as a family. They were now married and I had a new baby brother. We were 9 $1/2$ years old. I was his mom, I loved him and secretly whispered in his little earsthe day he came home from the hospital: "I will never let anything happen to you." I pretended he was my child.

My romance with alcohol began at the age of 13. The very first moment I took a sip of alcohol my world changed. A feeling of peace and warmth ran through my body, a peace I had never known. I felt beautiful, intelligent, calm and finally a part of this world. The feeling of being fat, ugly and unworthy all disappeared. I had found my new God. A God that would prove in the beginning to feel comforting and wonderful and an elixir that took away all the pain. This medication would only last for a short time until it became Satan, threatening my very being to its core.

Alcohol and addictions were not a stranger to my family. It was a history that was long and involved many generations. My grandparents were both alcoholics, my biological father, my uncle and my beautiful twin sister Diana; as well as many others. My family of origin was plagued with dysfunction, sickness and addictions. I guess my family was not abnormal compared to other families.

Diana went to University and studied Sociology. She worked a lot and finally got her degree in her field of study. I went to University and studied science. I wanted to become a Veterinarian. We were finally separated. Addictions took over our lives. We would come and go back to each other's place where ever we were living and it was alcoholic insanity.

At first I was a binge drinker. It was my medication and it made the world feel bearable. I didn't feel like the square peg trying to fit into a round hole anymore. Alcohol was my drug of choice, drinking in bars, alone, anywhere I could. I usually only drank on the weekends, worked all week and then repeated that cycle. The binges became closer and closer to the point when I lost everything. The police would pick me up many times and keep me in jail overnight for my safety. They would always say "what is a nice girl like you doing in a place like this?"

June 8th, 1992 was the beginning of my new life. At 29 years of age, I started treatment and graduated from a treatment centre. Living " One Day at a Time" practising the 12 Steps of Alcoholics Anonymous. By the grace of God, I have been able to remain sober since that date. Sobriety is not all pink roses. Life changes instantly. It is an everyday struggle and a lot of work. Getting authentic, having integrity, growing up and living life on life's terms.

My dear twin was not so fortunate. Di was in several treatment and detox centers. She didn't want to go to Alcoholics Anonymous or to see a psychiatrist as I had done for many years. Diana and I both suffered from major depressive disorder and severe anxiety. She refused to take any medication as it made her so sick and she would not seek professional help.

Drugs also crept into her life and she became addicted to Ativan. She never felt worthy about herself or loved herself and was always turning towards men that enabled alcohol consumption. Diana was always in competition with me and wanted the life I had created. She never had children of her own, however she had a very strong attraction to animals and created her own dog walking business.

The alcohol gradually took over more and more. I moved to Switzerland and married my husband who is from that country. Diana was very jealous of him and always said that he took me away from her. We had Diana live with us for a few months in Switzerland where I got her a job at the same place I worked at. When we were together everything was OK for about three days and then all hell would break loose. She needed to drink. The alcohol separated us. It tore us apart like nothing else ever had. We were different people now and we couldn't relate to one another anymore. Between my mom and myself we tried to help so much and it was very difficult and painful not being successful in our endeavors to help and see her this way. I loved her so much and I just wanted my sister back as we had been before.

My husband and I moved back to Canada where our two daughters were born. I somehow thought this would bring our family back together and that we would go to AA and Al-Anon together and everything would be well. A long time ago a psychiatrist told me that I was going to be the one to break the cycle of addiction and abuse in our family.

I kept loving my sister and I even made a point of going to Al-Anon. Even during her drinking times, I spoke to her regularly and I did not exercise the cardinal rule of "loving detachment or tough love" as taught in these programs. Our mother did, however, and she and Diana were always at war. It was too much for our mother to handle after what she had witnessed with her own very abusive alcoholic mother.

Thirteen years, prior, Diana had a very bad incident when the man she was dating beat her up so badly she nearly died. The police called me from Mount Sinai Hospital, and told me that my sister was there. She was in in rough shape when we finally got to see her and I almost did not recognize her. I was looking at this person so gone, beat up and in a very drunken and belligerent state, she was unrecognizable to me. The damage that was done to her head was so severe that I could see a portion of her brain. That was the moment I thought she would die. I thought this was it and she had finally hit rock bottom.

I really didn't know what to do at this point. As there was a waiting list for beds in that hospital, I decided to bring her home with us. I was going to take care of her again, fix her and make her whole. I thought she would live with us and everything would be the way it was when we were little. After three days however, she left again with a severe head injury and a desire to drink. During that time, victim services looked after her and the person who assaulted her was convicted and went to jail.

Diana moved once again and was looking for a geographical cure as she had done so many times in the past. As patterns repeat themselves, Diana once again attracted a man who became her drinking buddy and enabled her addictions. They stayed together for thirteen years.

Even during these trying times we talked to each other on a daily basis, we spoke about the beautiful times and all of the challenges ahead of us.

In conversations with my mother she always told me that Diana was going to die but I always insisted that I was going to fix her. She was in no shape to work, she was in a very depressive state and living on disability. I spoke to Diana every morning and every night depending on my work schedule. The one thing that Diana and I had always looked for was; approval, love and acceptance from our mother. Our mother always joked and said "she would not get the Mother of the Year award!!!" She harbored a lot of guilt and remorse for what had happened to us.

Diana started to have seizures and because of her substance abuse history the doctors called them pseudo seizures. Her doctor had put her on some medications for the seizures and Ativan for her severe anxiety.

Di was so energized and said that 2016 was going to be the best year ever. She always told me everything was okay, going well and not to worry. She planned to leave her partner after thirteen years and was going to start life all over again.

On January 28th, 2016 that all change at 7:55 p.m. when the doorbell was ringing at our home. I had not spoken to my sister that day after trying twice to call her. I felt something was very wrong. Everything was dull, dark and gloomy outside; I had a feeling the entire day that something was terribly wrong.

I thought who in this weather would be ringing the doorbell? My husband answered the door and I could only hear some men's voices. My first thought was that they were canvassing for something. My husband called me by my full name, which he never does, to come to the door. I got up and went around the corner and saw two Police Officers standing there. A chain of different thoughts went through my mind – my children, my mom, my car...? As I got closer I realized that it was Di. I grabbed my husband's arm and said 'No, please no, no!' They informed us that they received a report from the police department that Diana was found dead in her apartment. I had spoken to her the day before. I was going to work and she was so happy, this couldn't be true, no... I had to see her. They would not let me go and I didn't know where her body was. They took me to the couch as I was so sick - screaming, numb. I couldn't breathe and I did not believe them. My husband called my mother to deliver the tragic news.

Di was found 12 hours after she died. Her little dog Bentley was with her the entire time. Her partner found her after she did not show up for a meeting at the hospital. I tried to call that same morning to talk to her, no answer. I kept wondering if she was in pain, if she tried to cry out for help or get to a phone. I felt so distraught that she passed away all alone, only with her dog and I was not there to help her. When we entered her home to get her clothes and belongings, I laid where she had died for some time. I tried and tried to find her, to feel her and to smell her. She had just vanished. The room and her clothes were pristine and we could not even find any dirty laundry. I thought for sure she had harmed herself so she would no longer have to carry the pain. To say that I was completely out of my mind was an understatement. The coroner said that God's Angels came at 2:30 a.m. and took her away and that she did not feel anything and passed peacefully.

My heart was shattered into a million pieces. I thought that with half of me gone I am going to die as well. Twins do sometimes die close together and I was convinced that I was going go to sleep and die that evening as well.

During the visitation at the funeral home I thought I was going to see her and hold her for the last time. I brought a beautiful long mauve evening gown with a light purple pashmina shawl to keep her warm. I put my angels and books I had given her along the way with her beloved dog George's ashes into her coffin. They told us that we could not see her, that it would be a closed casket and that they had to remove several body parts, including her brain for the autopsy... I only had a casket with lace to hold on to.

The funeral was beautiful. On Monday at 1:00 p.m. the funeral home manager lit a candle and played music from Bette Midler's song "The Wind Beneath my Wings" as she walked behind the casket. Di had always told me that she wanted to be cremated because she was claustrophobic and afraid of being in the casket buried in the ground.

I also have experienced survival guilt. Why did she have to die first? Twin grief is very misunderstood. The surviving twin doesn't know how to move on in the beginning and feels a deep loss. The issue of identity can be an issue for identical twins as well as can abandonment and I felt both. Personal loss sent me into a profound deep sense of disconnection of who I was supposed to be now and how to live this "new normal." I kept thinking of my children, my husband, my animals as well as my other family members; I must go on.

The end of life for the surviving twin feels like the end of our lives forever. Life stopped for me, changed; and has never been the same since that moment. I feel life has not gone on since. I keep trying to find Di in the mirror, her voice on a tape or an answering machine a phone or a video. I called her so many times praying she would pick up. I was crazy with grief. I would put on her clothes on and refused to wash anything because everything smelled like her. At moments I would collapse, scream and yell at God for taking her from me.

I now had to learn how to be an "I" instead of a "we." I just didn't know how, it was not supposed to be this way. I felt half of me had been taken away, I was not whole anymore and I felt so vulnerable, very alone even when surrounded by many people.

I have started the painful journey of finding myself and who I am. The part inside of me that is missing, is so vast and I do not know how to fill that hole. There are no drugs, food, alcohol or magic relief that can ever replace it or fill that void.

The biological imprint of my twin will never leave me. Di is in my body, my heartbeat, my psyche and I am clinging to the shadows of my dearest departed sister in the physical being. The sense of separation is very painful but love does not die and in love there is no separation. Just like a sunbeam can't separate itself from the sun and a wave cannot separate itself from the ocean we will always be together until we meet again my love.

On April 27th, 2016 the coroner called us and in a very kind and empathetic voice. He told me that my beautiful twin's death was an accident. She suffered a grand malseizure and rolled over and suffocated in her pillow. Diana was drug fee however, there where traces of alcohol found in her body.

The disease of alcoholism and severe trauma steals many lives. It is not about will power or being strong it is about surrender and living life on life's terms.

Diana, I love you more than life itself. Until we meet again. The soul and spirit always carry on. There is so much grief because there was so much love– your other half, Adriane.

> Diana,
> I wrote your name in the sky,
> But the wind blew it away.
> I wrote your name in the sand,
> But the waves washed it away.
> I wrote your name in my heart,
> And forever it will stay.
> ~Jessica Blake

Sonia Commisso

My Beautiful Pathetic Life

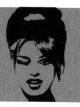

My life consisted of perfection. I had what I thought was a charmed life. I moved to the right area and sent my children to the right schools. I had a big house, nice cars, amazing friends and vacation after vacation. My life as I would call it was like a Christmas card. Everyone looking so perfect - just like a Christmas card. I look back and remember that it would take me weeks to find the right wardrobe so my family could match for our annual Christmas card. I was so "on" all the time as I call it. It was exhausting. As I look back I realize I was so judgmental, flawed and superficial. Being "on" was a full time job. The gossiping, clichés, drama, and exclusive memberships to clubs was exhausting.

My whole life I've been blessed. I succeeded in my educational goals and always got the jobs in the media industry. Major TV stations, successful advertising agencies and major tele-communication companies were some of my jobs. More recently I would been interviewing for various reality shows and I even landed a few of them. I lived a charmed life and always succeed at all my goals. Everything came easy to me because I looked the part - especially in the media industry which could sometimes be cruel. I was the epitome of society's obsession with the blonde hair, blue eyed Barbie-doll look. Between my looks and my career in media, I was successful and I felt successful. Then my first tragedy hit me when my father

199

died suddenly 24 years ago. I eventually went to work with my family and ended my media career. I got married, had three children and worked in the family business.

My famous saying to my 3 children (2 girls and a boy,) was "never be ordinary!" My spiritual journey began when my world fell apart one summer - my 19-year-old daughter went missing. My beautiful life became sad and pathetic very quickly. My life was so painful and broken into a million pieces that I sunk into a bottomless pit of despair with no way out. The pain I experienced was so extreme and unbearable. I thought it was difficult to cope when my father died suddenly, but my daughter missing was beyond any pain any human should suffer. When my dad died we had no control, it was the course of life that couldn't be prevented. My world fell apart and came crashing down when my daughter left. My awakening was very painful. I never looked at my true self until I discovered the answer through my journey, or as I call it, the loudest awakening of my life!

My oldest daughter proved that to me one summer. I would consider that the summer of my "awakening", the transformation that shook me to the core. My daughter decided to date a man 10 years her senior that had a criminal record. He was an unsavory character that no mother would have wanted her daughter to be with. He wasn't her knight in shining armor. As part of a large Italian family, it was impossible for my husband and I to approve of this relationship.

Instead, our mission was to destroy it. So we set out to do just that - or at least thought we could. With forty-five family members and friends, we tried to accomplish the impossible. We worked hard at this goal every day. Everyone had a role in the demise of this man. We worked hard to eliminate him from the equation. I'm not proud of this as I look back and reflect on what went down. I couldn't see past my hatred towards him. The end result was that my daughter left.

As painful as that was, it was my awakening. Living my life not knowing where she was for five months was beyond any pain a person should experience. Everyone was affected – mainly my other two children. They suffered in silence as they watched their mother and father turn into people they could not recognize anymore.

My house became a made for TV movie. Between police officers, social workers, private eyes I hired, family, friends and neighbors, I had no peace. I then realized I had to remove myself from the drama of this movie and start getting strong and in control of my life. Therapists, social workers, police officers, doctors, family and friends could not give me relief from my pain and suffering. My mind raced to deep dark places thinking of my daughter. The nights were brutally painful. I would think to myself, 'Is she dead or alive? Who is she with? What is she doing?' I would go in her bedroom and try to get one last scent of her through a perfume or clothing she wore. I remember sleeping in her bed and crying all night. Every time I went to sleep I would wish I wouldn't wake up because I couldn't handle the grief.

My grief was unbearable which made my panic attacks and anxiety worse. I remember grocery shopping and going by the fruit department and having a panic attack when

I saw strawberries and mangos (my daughter's favorite fruits.) I couldn't breathe. I fell to the ground and I don't remember anything except waking up in a hospital from the anxiety. Just looking at the fruit made me physically sick – again, a reminder of her missing.

The stress of setting the table for four people instead of five was so painful that I had to stop making dinner that summer because it triggered my anxiety. There was no relief from the pain. Everyone in the family felt the loss of my daughter, including my sister's dog. His ritual was to run to her room to play. After my daughter went missing, every time he came over he continued to look for her but eventually her scent went away and he stopped running upstairs for her. That vivid recollection makes me sad till this day.

I wanted to be induced to a coma state and wake up when it was over. All I kept hearing from people is that you have to carry on for your other two children. It felt like noise in my brain. Every time I tried, the situation just went from bad to worse. I'll never forget our first dinner as a family at a restaurant with just the four of us. My son had graduated from elementary school and won an award so we were determined to celebrate his victory, which was only fair to him. I froze and could not bring myself to walk in the restaurant with just the four of us. Everything in my body felt empty. I ran out crying. The whole restaurant experience was very traumatic.

I was on a course of self-destruction. I wanted my pain to stop. I hit rock bottom. I just couldn't do my life anymore and I struggled with myself and my identity. Feeling guilty as a mother and blaming myself for everything that went wrong, I spent every day thinking about the 'could haves' and the 'should haves.' I replayed that night over and over again. I felt guilty that I had failed my daughter. I wondered, if I had been more supportive, would she have left so abruptly? Everything was so mishandled and out of control.

The power struggle between my daughter and I raced through my mind all day. The conflict between us was so severe; it felt like there was no repairing the situation. My daughter tried to assert control of her life and I kept trying to control her. I always viewed her as my baby and not a woman. I was so angry and felt defeated. I tried to control everything and do all the right things but there was no right. Reasoning with her and providing logical arguments as to why this would be the biggest mistake of her life just brought out more hostility in her to the point where there could be no resolve. Growth is painful and with it comes a lot of agony.

Then my spiritual journey began. Slowly, with help from trained professionals, listening to their wise words and keeping a journal, I was able to pick myself out of my dark place and the process began. It started with the police officer who promised he would take away my pain. He patiently sat with me on a weekly basis and changed my way of thinking. He trained me on how to deal with her if and when I saw her again. How I would have to approach her and the words I needed to get through my first meeting with her. This filled my life with hope. Hope is what got me through my darkest times.

The first meeting did come and we had an encounter. She was sitting on a bench and I went up to her and said, "Hi." She looked up at me and I told her I loved her and asked if I could sit beside her and give her a hug. She looked at me and started to cry. She said "Yes, mom you can hug me and sit beside me." She looked like my baby girl again. So sad and confused just like when she was a child. All the words just began to flow from there. That first meeting lead to forty more meetings with her. Every meeting got easier and easier. It became my full time job to reintegrate her back into my life. This became my life mission for several months. It was a work in progress. Every text, every meeting was always on the hope that I would see her again. It was an emotional roller coaster every time I met with her.

My healing process began by forgetting about the past in order to move forward. I learned to love unconditionally and to leave my ego out of the equation. I chose my words very carefully at every encounter with her. I stopped being judgmental and learned not to discriminate. Remember, I lived in this perfect world where I created my own membership. That means in my world, the right house, clothes, cars, parties and friends. Membership was often denied if you didn't fit the profile. I saw the world through my eyes not my heart. This means when I started opening my eyes along with my heart and not being judgmental I found my spiritual side. This was pivotal to me in my awakening because I realized when you look into a person's soul, life looks a lot different.

When I found my soul I was reborn. My ego didn't exist anymore and my judgmental side died. My cliché life where membership could be denied unless you lived in that

"Christmas card" world was expired. I was no longer that girl that looked for faults in others by gossiping and being shallow. I finally see people for who they are and the soul that is attached to them. I was awakened and I began to embrace my daughter and all her amazing qualities that made her the strong person she had become and the spectacular young lady she is going to be – even though some of her choices broke my heart. Sometimes coming to terms with reality is difficult. That's why I learned that the small victories win the war. I won the war because my daughter became part of my life again. It took time and patience and a lot of love.

I became Sonia 2.0. The old Sonia 1.0 was gone. I was like a new improved iPhone and my pathetic life started to look beautiful again. My therapist taught me that you need to "get shot before you bleed." I was always bleeding before I got shot. Which in my world meant that I wrote the script before it played out. I have learned to deal with the situation in the moment it is presented to me and not worrying about the future. My daughter still hasn't come home, but I've learned detachment love through this path. I can still love her from a distance and embrace our not so perfect relationship and accept her decisions even though I don't agree with them all. My daughter's path is her own to live – without judgment and without conditions.

I embrace my daughter because this is her journey and growth to womanhood. All her morals and values are intact and she is amazing. We have both changed and we came out on the other side. I respect her as a woman and she respects me as her mother. Parenting doesn't come with a manual.

Sonia 2.0 realized in her journey that a lot of people may be beautiful to look at but they aren't authentic. I only wanted to show the world beauty, which made me lose touch with what was truly important. I was that superficial person caught up in the drama and gossip. I realized my behavior wasn't allowing me to live my authentic self. I wasn't being true to myself and my tragedy has allowed me to embrace the beauty in myself and see the beauty in others. I'm a better person after this struggle. My situation enlightened my whole life and put it into perspective. The values I held true in the past are no longer my truth. I've learned to accept myself with all my faults and strengths in my beautiful and not so pathetic life.

Samantha King

Work/Life Balance:
The Holy Grail of Womanhood

You don't know me, but trust me when I say that I'm not one to beat around the bush. With that in mind, I'm going to get straight down to the heart of the matter. The idea of work/life balance, as we know it, is a myth.

This is a story about how I came to that conclusion.

But first I want to paint a picture for you. I want you to think about each of these things: The Holy Grail. The Lost City of Atlantis. Let's throw in the Fountain of Youth too, while we're at it. At the end of the day, they're all things that many characters of myth dedicated and risked their lives to find, but that were only accessible to a select few. As a woman in today's world, trying to balance career, family and everything in between, I've spent a lot of time feeling that the idea of work/life balance was just another one of these myths. I would chase it tirelessly, but it seemed that only a select few could ever reach it... and I wasn't one of them - no matter how hard I tried.

What was making me feel this way? Simple. Social media. In today's world, there is no end to the number of ways we can connect with others and peek "behind" the curtains of their lives. And, to be honest, their lives usually look... great. They're always smiling, hitting exciting milestones — either personally or professionally, out doing fun stuff with their kids, or just enjoying the moments around them. No wonder I felt like this coveted way of life was for everyone but me. However, if you looked at my life online five years ago, you might have thought I was one of the select few... because, honestly, who puts the dark and twisty parts of life online?

Here's what was actually happening...

I was a hot mess that had hit rock bottom. It was June 2015. A short 6 weeks earlier, my daughter, Penny, then four, had been diagnosed with autism after 18 months of playing, what I like to call, the 'Is she or isn't she?' game with the many professionals we encountered as we tried to get help for our child. To say that my world was upside down and swirling as I tried to wrap my head around the diagnosis and figure out the next steps for Penny was an understatement. What's more,I had just given birth to my second child, Max.

Three days after his birth, we were heading to visit family when a wave of anxiety more severe than I had ever felt washed over me. The need to escape and get out of the car was so strong that I seriously considered jumping out of the moving vehicle. And that was just the beginning.

As the sun set, I began to stress out over the idea of night-time. To this day I can't quite explain it. Whether it was the loneliness, perception of nowhere to run to as everything stopped, or just the eerie quiet, I can't say. What I do know is that I spent that entire night feeling on edge. There seemed to be nothing I could do to "take my mind off it." My body alternated between feelings of nausea, tingling sensations running throughout it, and an overall inability to sit still for more than a minute or two. My mind was filled with a combination of irrational thoughts and fear at those thoughts. It was almost like an out-of-body experience. I knew on some level that the thoughts that were inundating my mind made no sense, but I had no control or ability to stop them. Essentially, I felt like I was losing my mind.

I was lucky though. I had a supportive husband, a great family doctor, and some experience with postpartum depression from after Penny's birth. The coming weeks were filled with more of the symptoms from that first night, along with some additional - and equally emotional - feelings. It got to the point where I spent most of my days and nights pacing unable to quiet the thoughts in my mind to a point where I felt safe enough to stop...or get any sleep. I couldn't stand holding my newborn son or having to deal with Penny and her needs. I hovered around my husband constantly trying to gain some sense of security. I even waited outside the washroom door like a toddler until he came out; the entire time dreading the possibility that one of my children would try to interact with me or need something from me. When I wasn't doing that, I was so depressed that I couldn't be bothered to get out of bed, and, if I did get out bed, I was visibly detached and zoned out watching episodes of Paw Patrol (I still can't watch that show without reliving the whole experience all over again).

With the help of medications, counseling and frequent visits from medical professionals, I slowly regained my ability to cope and, over the following months, to function. Eventually, I was able to connect with my son and reconnect with my life, but the anxiety and depression are things I still struggle with every single day.

When you hit rock bottom, you inevitably reflect on your life as you try to climb your way out...

As I mentioned, this wasn't my first time in the ring with postpartum depression. After Penny's first birthday, anxiety forced me to leave my supply teaching position because I just couldn't get into the classrooms. Here I was again, three years later, in the same spot... but even worse. Now, I was facing depression, disconnect and an anxiety that was far worse than anything I had ever faced before.

As I worked to come out of the dark and twisty hole I felt myself living in, I started to reflect on what my life looked like up until now. At 31 years old, I realized that I had never taken the time to figure out what I wanted out of life. Where was it all going?

Upon completion of high school, I pursued a post secondary degree on the basis of, "I might as well study something I like." When I was done with that degree, I went on to Teacher's College and continued down a path that had me sitting here in the present day – 31 years old with experience in four different industries since leaving university at age 24. Don't get me wrong. I learned a lot in each position and field, but I had never had any real sense of where I was going. From the outside, it sure looked like I had a plan. I was successful at each job I took, but the reality was much different. My success was more the result of natural ability, quick learning and self starting, and sheer workaholism. All great qualities (okay, maybe not the workaholism), but, without a plan, there was a lot of start and stops that, if I was being honest, had really led me nowhere. I was essentially no further ahead than the day I left university, and it was a tough pill to swallow.

What was even more alarming was that during this reflection, nothing even registered outside of my career. Nothing about my own personal development, my marriage, or my kids. They didn't even come into the equation. (I said I was a workaholic, didn't I?) I'm not saying that these areas of my life weren't fine, but how much better could they be if I spent some time actually figuring out what I wanted from them and what I needed to do to get there? That thought had the wheels turning.

After those months of reflection, I was pumped. I don't know if it was the counseling, the relief and fog lifting after hitting rock bottom, or that I am a creative person who thrives off new ideas, but I was ready to jump feet first into a complete change of lifestyle. Thankfully the people around me were excited, supportive, and... cautious. It was lovingly pointed out to me that, given my fragile mental state, I needed to take my time in this new phase of my life. I needed to crawl before I could walk. While time, counseling and medications had given me a renewed sense of hope and purpose, like the recovery to anything else, too much too soon was a real problem.

We've all heard that adage 'a place for everything and everything in its place,' and that's how we all seem to naturally try to organize our lives. So, I was not surprised that this was the overwhelming recommendation of those around me when helping me get started. I slowly began to create structure in my day-to-day life. I began following a strict routine where everything had its own time and place, which was also very helpful for Penny as we tried to navigate this new world of autism. And, while that was a big part of how I was able to come back to the land of the living, before I knew it, maternity leave was ending and I was going to have to add another factor into the mix – one that I wouldn't be in control of – work.

The Biggest Hurdle This Workaholic Had To Overcome...

As women, we are pulled in a million different directions based on whatever is screaming the loudest — sometimes that's our career/business; sometimes it's our marriage; sometimes it's other areas of our personal life... for me, it's usually my two children, as I am the primary caregiver, followed closely by my workaholic tendencies.

When it was time to go back to work, I began thinking about what my life had been like prior to having Max. My husband works off hours leaving me feeling like a single parent most days. I was sleep deprived as the result of keeping weird hours. Shuttling Penny back and forth between daycare, assessments and therapy sessions; grabbing food as I raced along, and then getting a little time with her through the dinner chaos, homework from therapy, and bedtime fights. When she was finally in bed (not asleep... just in bed), I would take out my laptop to "finish up a few things" while binge watching whatever looked good on Netflix. Three hours later, I was asleep on the couch only to wake up exhausted in a few short hours to do it all over again. I felt like Bill Murray in Groundhog Day.

With Penny's newly cemented diagnosis, and the lack of a road map where her care was concerned (I'm still flying blind two years later), I couldn't go back to that life. I had been lucky in my last position that my employers were family oriented people, who were willing to let me make up time from home on evenings and weekends when Penny's therapy sessions called for me to be out of the office once a week for eight weeks straight. I can honestly say that is not the norm for parents of children with special needs who have to work in order to support their children's care. With a formal diagnosis, there would be even more sessions. Additionally, she was entering school now, and that meant a whole new set of professionals to coordinate and work with. It also meant having to be available should she have a meltdown and need to be picked up from school when the environment became too much for her senses to handle now that she didn't have a nap/quiet time in the afternoon to regroup. I was essentially unemployable in most employer's eyes... a path that all special needs parents inevitably have to cross in some way.

With the support of my family, and the good fortune that I was in a position that allowed me to, I started my own coaching business. As I did this, I tried to continue working with the 'a place for everything and everything in its place' approach to balancing the many things vying for my time. However, no matter how I hard tried, something always got dropped or left behind. The things that I wanted at the top of the list were never at the top, and, if I spent all day working on one area, then three other areas would get backed up. At the end of the day, I was left frustrated, overwhelmed, angry and, above all else, feeling incapable and guilty.

So I began thinking...

Here I was on a mission to help female entrepreneurs build their dreams while creating the work/life balance they craved, and I could barely keep my own head above water. Not ready to hit rock bottom again, I started to question why this was the prevailing way society suggests we try to achieve work/life balance. And, while I have yet to figure out the answer, what I do know is that for me (and many of the women I know) it doesn't exist in two distinct, clear cut realms. It's not one or the other for us. It's not work or life. It doesn't even look the same from day-to-day, for that matter. So why were we trying to achieve it this way? No wonder we were ripping our hair out.

I'm not saying that work/life balance doesn't exist. It absolutely can exist... just not the way we are envisioning it. I realized that if we keep trying to achieve work life/balance through this 'everything has its time and place' approach, we're never going to have it. At the end of the day, it is always going to end up being the coveted treasure that women are constantly chasing, struggling to get right, and then feeling guilty when they don't.

This pissed me off too.

The departments of my Fempire

In that moment, the shift happened. The life I am building now no longer looks at work/life balance as a one or the other kind of deal. The 'a place for everything and everything in its place' philosophy was thrown out the window. My empire (I call it a Fempire) is more than just my career, and I'm not the only woman in this boat. I stopped thinking about my Fempire as just my business and began thinking about it as my legacy. A legacy that had many different components centered around the many different areas of my life.

Never able to truly let go of my workaholism, I began to structure my new norm the same way I would structure a business – including each area of my life that would make up my legacy as a department within my Fempire. There is a department for Penny, now 6, and all of her needs. I've got a department for Max, my 2 year old car fanatic with a speech delay and his own set of professionals and therapies to help him work through that. And I've got a department for myself, my husband and all of our shared goals, and, of course, one for my actual business. Each department has its own lists of projects and priorities, which helps me keep everything straight. However, unlike before, I don't keep each department separated with its own time and space dedicated to it, as if in those places and moments are the only times I can work on them. That's not how you a run a business. That's not how I'm running this business.

As the CEO of this business, I have a team of trusted, capable professionals/partners that I work with who I have to delegate to and lean on for support. Because, as the CEO, I can't focus on only one department at a time or lose sight of where each department stands presently vs. where it needs to stand 6 months from now. So I manage each department simultaneously by prioritizing them all collectively.

What does that mean? It means one collective list of tasks organized by priority sprinkled throughout my week. It means appointments for me scheduled in between meetings and calls during the day because that's when I have care for my kids. It means working a little on the weekends while Max naps so I can be around to take Penny or Max to therapy throughout the week.

By being clear about what each department is and what it needs, I have a constant checklist as I go into every week that allows me to easily get a handle on what needs to be done. From there, I go through my checklist of departments and make sure that I schedule in a task or two to keep each department moving forward. I know where each department stands, and am able to confidently say that nothing is getting dropped.

Today my office is my happy place where my daughter has a desk to work at, my son plays on the floor, and I've got The Big Bang Theory playing in the background while I knock off business tasks. Tomorrow I might spend more time shuttling them around and refereeing the two of them instead. But that's what true balance is - because life doesn't fit nice and neatly into allotted times. What I'm working on and what balance looks like for me changes from day-to-day. It's a constant work in progress, but, as I long as I know that I am moving each department forward and building that legacy, I'm happy. Sure, people may think that it's going to take longer for me to get to the end goal, but I can rest easy at night knowing that, slowly but surely, I will get where I've decided I want to go... in a way that both myself and my family can be proud of.

Amy Stockwell

6 Steps For Living Your Truth

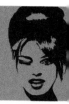

Question... Have you ever asked yourself, 'Is this all that there is? What now? Why bother? If only... Why aren't I enough? Am I lovable?'

If you are courageous enough to say yes to any of the above questions, you rock for being honest – and welcome to the human race. You are not alone. I have asked myself those questions over and over again for many years as I felt stuck and in a negative funk a lot of the time. Joy would come and it would easily go – it never seemed to stay. I was full of self-doubt to the point that I couldn't trust myself to make a decision and I judged everything I said or did. I asked for other's opinions of what was best for me over my own thinking. I never felt good enough or lovable, or looked at myself as a worthwhile person – and I wondered why joy wouldn't stay the night with me? Yikes! Yes, I was that person that people were afraid to ask the simple question, "'how are you?", because after I said "fine" came a brief pause and then a laundry list of what was going wrong in my life! That was my negative thinking taking over and it was a buzz kill! I could only try and keep myself afloat for so long until ultimately I hit rock bottom. It could have gone 2 ways, up – or further down into more empty ice cream cartons with extra self-loathing on top! My life became so unmanageable that I was finally willing to do anything to get out of this negative vortex!

My way out was to start a quest. I needed to get answers to those questions I kept asking myself repeatedly, with the ultimate goal of feeling good within myself. It wasn't easy, but it was very worth it. I had to learn who I was, how I thought about things, how my actions and reactions were affecting my joy and then develop new behaviors that would serve me better. As you can tell, I like using humor too, it helps. I had to take a real honest look at myself and my flaws to see what was tripping me up in life. The vicious cycle of the routine song and dance of anxiety – short burst of joy – depression – short burst of joy – more anxiety – short burst of joy – self-pity-fear-short burst of joy - oh look – ice cream! It was a rollercoaster of emotions that started from the time I was a child until the time I hit rock bottom in my early thirties. You can only run from yourself and your problems for so long, have so many comebacks from sorrow, until you get tired and give up and settle on life. I was very close to that, but this time I was so exhausted and did not have much mojo left!

Like an epic concert moment that you are in disbelief that you are experiencing, rock bottom came to town the fall of 2013 with the headliner being my marriage ending. Everything seemed to happen all at once as my employer suggested that I take some time off because they were concerned about my well being and job performance. In disbelief I said, "I'm fine" - no twenty-minute complaint session that I subjected my poor colleagues to at the copier machine, just disbelief that the meeting with my supervisor was not what I expected. On top of it all my children were acting out – and rightly so, as we had moved in with my mother in her small three-bedroom bungalow. Everyone's world had been rocked – but not in the epic best concert of your life kind of way. Wow, I felt stellar about myself... Not! It just seemed that everything around me had become so unmanageable and I was the only one oblivious to it. But when denial slaps you in the face there is no hiding from it anymore. My mom would often say "you need to listen to the universe when it's tapping you gently on the shoulder not bitch slapping you." Thank you, Mom, I found that one out the hard way!

At first it was tough hearing what my Mom had to say because most of my life I really resented her. I grew up in an alcoholic home as my dad was a drinker. Domestic violence was part of my dysfunctional upbringing. On top of that I was sexually abused at the age of five. When I was nine years old, my mom, older sister and I were removed from our home by child protection services and lived in a shelter for about six months. We finally got our own place and my mother did not know what else to do but work. This created a lot of resentment as I felt so abandoned by my parents.

That theme of abandonment carried through my entire life, guided my decisions, behaviors, and the choices that I made, although at the time I was not aware of this. By the time all this dysfunction came crashing down when I was 31 years old, it was the Universe saying, "Girl, get your damn-ass demons sorted out and get on with your life." To me, for some reason, the voice of the universe is a boisterous African American woman, saying things straight up, with soul. Thus, hitting rock bottom was really a time to heal my emotional wounds so I could start living life like I never had before – full of hope, wonder, and excitement!

I think my red-carpet, award winning moment in my breakdown came when I was in the grips of my depression, about a month into living at my moms'. One morning I emerged from my room the picturesque depiction of depression; uncombed hair, the yoga pants I wore for four day stretches at a time that conveniently converted into pajamas, no bra (going on the fifth or sixth day in a row), and puffy red eyes from crying over a man who couldn't give me the love I needed. My mom greeted me with coffee (my only joy at this point), as I shuffled into the kitchen. The kids were eating their breakfast and talking about some funny show. Somehow I could find a way to make it sad and cry, and I was just so fed up with feeling like crap. I looked at my mom and said, "I can't, Mom. I give up, why bother? I'm broken. I'll never be lovable. Why wasn't I enough for him? How is my life going to get better?"

She looked at me and said, "Amy, God gives his toughest battles to those who are strong enough to handle them." "Really? I said, "Either this is some kind of sick joke God is laughing at or he must think I'm Joan-of-f#@king-Arc because this is too tough!" My mom hugged me and said, "Just get the kids to school and come back home to cry." This was just cruel and unusual punishment, I thought to myself. What the heck did I do so bad to deserve this? Was my childhood not crappy enough that now God was punishing me even further with some sick and twisted game of 'how much crap can Amy handle in one life'? Like, come on!

I eventually realized that no, this wasn't a sick game and the Universe wasn't punishing me. It led me to work on myself, allowing me to grieve and reach the conclusion that the Universe doesn't punish or get its kicks from seeing others suffer (or seeing how many outfits they can make out of one pair of over worn yoga pants!) That's not how it works. The Universe saves your ass with these painful lessons if you are so daring as to acknowledge yourself. My therapist and mentor gave me these steps to help me see that everything in my life leading up until now, even as I type this, is a result of my choices. Yes, we all have stress, unforeseen circumstances happen to us, things we did not plan on happening happen, and plot twists. But it is how we deal with these events and past experiences that shape our present. Below is the Adult State of Mind, the steps I used to guide myself out of depression, letting go of a lifetime of negativity.

#1. I Am Responsible For Me Only. No Blame.

Every thought/feeling I own. You get to be you. I get to be me. No one can make me feel, or to feel. I have to have a thought first. Read that over. No one can make you feel. How many times have you said to someone "you're making me feel like ____." They're not! You are. Because as I tell my children, no one can make them feel – because no one is your head and no one is your heart. People can impact you totally. But how you perceive things and respond with your behavior is your call.

#2. I Am Accountable For Me. No More Tit For Tat.

No more "Well you did this,"; "Oh yeah? Well that's because you did this."

You know those arguments, like you're dealing with a five-year-old? Yeah – that's keeping score, and it only works in sports and with five-year-olds on playgrounds. Keeping score means all your energy is tied up in keeping a running tally of resentments. Like when you are driving to work and thinking about what others have done to you and then mentally compartmentalizing it, only to retrieve it when you go home and then explode on the person you care about the minute you walk through the door. This is where we rob ourselves of joy and the positive energy we could be feeling instead of keeping score. Let it go for you.

#3. No More "If Only's" – I Am Not A Victim.

If only they would change; if only you got the promotion; if only the renovation would be done; if only you had more money; if only they would see things exactly like you do… the list goes on and can be tailored to your preference. If only _____ would happen, then I would be happy.

Wrong! All this type of thinking does is keep you feeling like a victim. I thought this way for a very long time and it made me feel powerless – like I had no control or say with what goes on in my life. It makes a whole lot of sense if your happiness is contingent upon external forces and events needing to take place. You could be waiting your whole life! Some of these things may never happen and that's just the holy all

222

about that! Combine that with a victim mentality and your happiness may never happen either. Yikes! That is not going to fly. What you could do instead is to decide to be content today whether things in your life happen or not. You can also let go of the control. That was tough for me, but not impossible, just tough. When you admit what you are powerless over and realize the only thing in life you really can control is you, you will feel empowered. That is the polar opposite of feeling victimized. Don't put your happiness in the outcomes of people, places, and things

#4. I Am Dedicated To My Reality. I Know Who I Am. I Know You. I Know What I Know.

I didn't know myself for a long time and that was a big problem. The result was that I didn't know how to read myself and others. Therefore, I would often second guess myself and the situations I would find myself in. Looking back now, I don't believe people were trying to talk me out of what I knew as truth, I think they were just telling me how they saw things. Their perception. When I realized they were seeing things through their reality and I was seeing things through mine, I could just accept we saw things differently and that was okay. From that insight I stopped second guessing myself and sugar coating the realities unfolding all around me. Excuses for other people's behavior stopped, also for myself. I know me better than anyone, I know my truth better than anyone, and I know what to do to take care of myself better than anyone. Am I wrong sometimes? Absolutely, because I am not perfect. However, I do handle those mistakes much better than before and they do not happen as frequently now that I know myself!

#5. My Life Is Up To Me. What Am I Going To Do About It?

You know those awesome quotes about how the first chapter of your life may have gone a certain way, maybe not the best, but you can write the next chapter and ultimately the ending to your epic life story? This is what they mean. Stuff happens, the force of life happens, and there are things we just cannot control. So what am I going to do about it? I found that being willing to restore my faith in a power greater than myself, be it God, Mother Nature, or my late granny in heaven, there was a power greater than I working its magic and things in my life happened for a reason. With that acceptance I could then build up the courage to do something about my circumstances. I took responsibility for my life and stopped blaming the past or other people for my current misfortunes. When that sunk in, I could see that I needed to get into the driver's seat of my life because no one is going to care about my happiness more than me. So why did I spend so much time putting it into the hands of others?? As my Mom says, "when you know better, you do better." Now you can do the same!

#6. I Must Learn To Tell The Truth. I Must Learn To Say No.

Ewww! Ugh! Ick! What will others think if I tell them what is really on my mind? What if it upsets them? Oh and then there is the let down and guilt I will feel from saying no and disappointing them! Clearly, the best thing to do is to smile and nod; put other's feelings ahead of my own, and then gripe about it later in private. Not! But that is what I did for most of my life. No wonder I would feel bitter and resentful towards others. I learned early on to worry about other people's feelings more than my own, even if that meant lying and holding back from what I truly wanted to say, and needed to do to take care of myself. From years of doing that to myself I became restless and tired and decided enough was enough - I am going to be me. This meant being honest and direct in communicating my needs and views to others. This meant saying no when I needed to and not taking the responsibility for other's actions. When I started doing this, my self-esteem took a major boost because I felt empowered. Sometimes it can be tricky but not nearly like it was before I went to work on myself!

One of the hardest things in life was to get real with myself. Those six steps created a state of mind that helped me navigate the world while sorting myself out. I knew deep down before I started connecting with myself that my formula was not working. I would go in and out of joy and it would never last. I would second guess myself and value other's opinions of me and how to handle my problems more than my own self-efficacy! However, through some of the greatest storms in my life have come so much prosperity. You can't put a price on the gift of self-discovery and coming out of denial. That is the hardest part – to admit your baggage to yourself and then to have the courage to look at it and change it. With little steps taken daily there is hope. When my marriage ended and I was sent off from work it was devastating. Those times really made me call upon my inner strength and get resourceful. I did everything I could to work through the pain and not run from it like I always did. Joining a support group that I still attend, seeking out my mentor for therapy, creating new hobbies, reading self-development literature, and surrounding myself with people who allowed me to pick myself back up at my own rate and pace was the turning point for me. I continue the practices that got me out of a negative pattern because I believe life is a series of learning and things can be maintained. You can't cure self-doubt but you sure can manage it with self-esteem. You can't cure fear but you sure can manage it with love. As long as I continue to do the things that help me manage my life I can roll with the ups and downs because that is life. I obviously want more ups than downs, but I am that much more aware. I know it will be okay because there are solutions to my problems, and answers I am looking for. The end of the world is the end of the world, so until I am falling into a black hole from the ground beneath my feet, I've got this. My job is to prepare for joy. With my guiding steps that is possible. Dr. Norman Vincent Peale said, "an empty mind generates power." And when I live life from joy I empty my mind to carry on and keep going.

"And that's just the holy all about it," as my mom says!

Teresa Ursini

Know Thyself

I was silent for far too long. I was always being told to be quiet. 'Children should be seen and not heard,' had been constantly drummed into my head. I was told that no one should air their dirty laundry out in public. I needed to talk but so many times I stopped myself from telling a friend or family member what I was truly feeling. Early on, I developed an insecurity about my self-worth.

I felt completely alone, always suffering and stifled, not able to talk to anyone, or share what was going on in my mind. I really hoped and dreamed that my family would be different – my craving just to be "normal." What is normal? We make our own normal. I always wished my family would speak without arguing or being loud.

As a child, I would hear loud arguing so many nights – and it deeply affected me. I was scared and alone with only my radio in my room, I lay down on my bed, listening to music and the darkness of night.

As a family the only time we ever sat down for family dinners together was at Christmas and Easter. Even on important holidays like Christmas, only my mom and I put up the tree. It was disappointing that nobody else in our family felt it was as important as I did.

How I longed for that family time to just talk about anything. But instead, everyone ate quickly, and then ran out. There was never any time to chat or connect. It was mostly my mom and I eating by ourselves. I felt angry and disappointed that it was this way. It had been a frustrating and lonely time for me. The feeling of being unappreciated engulfed me. Escape was all I could think about and I was determined.

It wasn't just at home that I had experienced loneliness. School was also a place that I wanted escape from. I had been bullied and told I was ugly. Kids can be cruel. I had always wanted to be beautiful and successful. Driven by these thoughts, I found my inner strength and consciously decided to rise above all of the negative words and negative people around me.

Gone were the days of feeling afraid and unsure of myself! I embraced positive people into my life to help me achieve my goals. No more silence. No more fear. I aspired to have that peaceful home I had dreamed of a safe haven where I could be my true self.

This vision became my reality when I met my prince. He brought out the best in me. Finally, I was confident that I made the right choice to co-create the life I so desired. I became the person who I always was meant to be, using my voice and speaking out loud. How free I felt when I was able to talk about my feelings and express my inner lion, my inner warrior.

Yes, dreams do come true. I inherently knew that I deserved to be happy. My family that I created was everything I had wished for growing up. I had the loving husband, two children and successful career. We had dinner together every night and talked as a family. I made Christmas and Easter a very special family time. Putting up the Christmas tree together, having Easter hunts, making birthdays very special days. We had fun together, we laughed – and I encouraged my own family to speak about their inner feelings without judgment. My experiences as a child made me become a stronger adult, that is for sure.

Then – my perfect world that I had created shattered into a million pieces. That life changing day happened in 1989 when I was diagnosed with thyroid cancer.

My doctor called to say the results of my biopsy had come in after only two days. He needed to see me. I really thought nothing of it because I was only 32 years old and in good health. WRONG! Confident that all would be fine, I had brought my two children (ages 6 and 4) with me to get my results. That was a BIG MISTAKE!

My doctor started the conversation, "Would you like the good news first or the bad news?", he paused.

"What bad news?" I quickly replied.

He continued, "You have thyroid cancer, it's a small nodule. I think we caught it in time. Once we remove the nodule we will know more. I have scheduled you at the hospital for surgery Friday to remove it."

"WHAT!?" I was stunned. I looked at my two little babies standing there looking at me. The fear set in.

"DOCTOR, WHAT DID YOU SAY?" I couldn't believe what he was telling me.

The doctor tried to set my mind at ease, "Well, if you're going to get cancer, thyroid cancer is the best one to get, it grows very slowly."

I stared at him in disbelief. "No cancer is a good cancer in my opinion."

On auto-pilot, I put the kids in the car and proceeded to drive home. In hindsight, I realized I shouldn't have driven by myself with the kids in the car. I should have called my husband - or anybody to come and pick me up. I was trying to be strong for the children's sake, but I just couldn't contain myself. Five minutes into the car ride, I started crying to the point that I could not even speak. I must have had a guardian angel on my side, because I have no idea how I even made it home.

My son was yelling, "MOMMY... MOMMY... WHY ARE YOU CRYING?"

My daughter putting her arms around her little brother, said, "MOMMY JUST GOT SOME BAD NEWS". She was 6 years old going on 16. Through the rear view mirror I witnessed my daughter reach out to her brother. It touched me so much that I cried even more. I couldn't believe what I had done. My daughter had understood everything the doctor was telling me. I was so angry at myself. Why didn't I go to the doctor's office with my husband?

Playing it all back in my mind, I truly never thought there would be anything wrong with my health. I heard shattered glass in my head and I felt the shards cutting my heart. Immediately, I thought – 'who will take care of my children?' I thought of my Prince. My husband. We had been married for only 10 years. I had been a very happy, social person that had everything I dreamed of. Now, what?

This is when the panic and anxiety set in. I had never felt anxiety before. This was panic attack anxiety. It truly felt like I was having a heart attack. I was petrified. Tears began pouring out.

On one particular day, my anxiety reached its peak. I had been grocery shopping and it hit me so hard. I had to get out of there! Abruptly, I bolted for the door, leaving a full shopping cart of groceries in the aisle. I couldn't wait to get home. That afternoon, I couldn't stop crying. Between the tears and the fear I thought I would never get back to my normal self. My mind was swirling. The thought of not being there to watch my children grow was devastating.

I opened up and told my husband my deepest and darkest feelings, shared my fears and pain. He gave me the biggest hug and said "We will do this together." Darn Cancer. With that support, I felt assured that we absolutely could beat this together.

As the treatment continued, the doctors were confident that they got all the cancer out. I felt a huge sense relief until I was given a 5-year window. If it doesn't come back in the next 5 years then you're okay. All I have to do is to take thyroid medication for the rest of my life, but that is fine. I AM ALIVE.

Now, the time was ticking. 5 years. Wow – 5 years of this hanging over my head. The constant fear, in the back of my mind. Over those 5 years my anxiety grew worse. I felt I needed to help myself deal with this nightmare just as I did back in my childhood.

I felt completely alone – but I knew I wasn't alone. I read so many self-help books. I discovered that many other people also suffered from terrible anxiety. This truly helped me. I realized that I wasn't alone. I turned my dark thoughts around and always looked for the "light ." Music which had always been my savior, soothed my inner spirit and soul. It was and always will be my drug of choice.

This journey allowed me to speak out loud. I started to turn to family and friends. I couldn't be quiet about my inner feelings any longer. I realized that, being silent is a cancer in itself. I say it out loud so I don't feel the anxiety of my fears anymore.

Life is a precious gift: I want to live my life to the fullest, and I do. It is full of obstacles but I believe it's how we choose to deal with each and every obstacle one step, one day at a time. Live in the present, live in the light and always be true to yourself.

Self Acceptance

"Have patience with all things but first with yourself.
Never confuse your mistakes with your value as a
human being.
You're a perfectly valuable creative worthwhile person
simply because you exist.
No amount of triumphs or tribulations can ever
change that.
Unconditional self – acceptance is the core of a
peaceful mind."
~Robert U

"relentless and the endless pursuit of light"
~Alan Frew

Live Out Loud is a beautifully vulnerable collection of stories that speak to our deepest fears, let us know we are not alone, and inspire hope that no matter what has happened in the past we can take charge of our futures and become the women we are meant to be. There truly is something here for everyone."
~Tara Bradford, Huffington Post Contributor

The Sisterhood ƒolios is precisely one of those books that has healing power in every word. These brave, beautiful women share their raw and real stories of struggle that every human being can resonate with at some level. I found it inspiring to read that each of these courageous souls found the power and wisdom within them that we ALL have access to. If you are craving your own personal transformation or simple human connection that will touch your heart... it lies within the pages of The Sisterhood ƒolios.
~Michelle Dunk, In beTWEEN Girls

The Sisterhood ƒolios: Live Out Loud is a compilation of stories that women have experienced and how the experiences shaped them into the women they are today.
~Laura Starner, Cheerleader of Hope

Live Out Loud made me laugh and cry. Every woman has a story. A lot of us are scared to share our story because we think we will be judged. But when we share our story we give someone else validation and acceptance. A reader can see themselves in that same scenario and realize they're not alone. Someone else understands them. Well, that's exactly what happened when I read this book. I could see myself in every one of these stories of triumph and overcoming major fears and obstacles! I just couldn't put it down.
~Linda Hayles, Huffington Post contributor

We're often hurt, confused or misguided, and life throws us curve balls, yet we're always striving for stronger, deeper satisfaction and happiness – and as a whole, these essays make that goal seem fully possible.
~ Julie Bookman, Books for Kids, The Atlanta Journal–Constitution

WHAT IS YOUR STORY?

Have you ever said, "I should write my story"?

Is writing a book on your Bucket List?

Do you realize, that by sharing your journey,
you are helping yourself and others?

Impart your wisdom and make a difference!

This will give you a taste for writing
without the pressure of an entire book!

**Are you ready to write your own book?
We also do SOLO AUTHOR projects.**

More volumes coming in
The Sisterhood *folios*:

The first volume in
Women Think Business –

Born to be Me   **Ingite your
Inner Warrior**

The Balancing Act

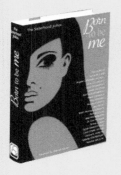 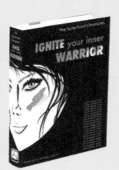 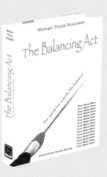 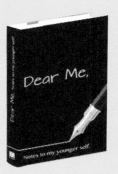

Dear Me – **Notes to my Younger Self**
Experiences, thoughts and lessons
I wish I could share with my younger self.

Inquire about contributing a chapter.

info@creativepublishinggroup.com
www.creativepublishinggroup.com

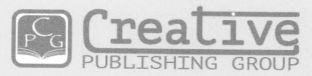

CPSIA information can be obtained
at www.ICGtesting.com
Printed in the USA
LVOW05s0427160917
548559LV00010B/25/P

9 780995 881037